ROBERT FALCONER-TAYLOR
PETER NEVILL
VAL STRONG

Intelligence

The EMRA™ Approach to Pet
Behaviour Problem Assessment and
Treatment

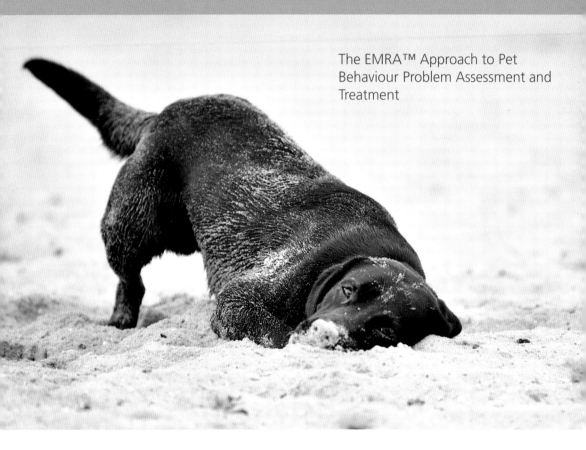

 CENTRE OF APPLIED PET ETHOLOGY (COAPE)
Partners and main authors:
Robert Falconer-Taylor, Peter Neville, Val Strong
COAPE-diplomats and authors of the case histories:
Hannah Lyon, Billie Machelle, Kirsty Peake and Alison Rengert

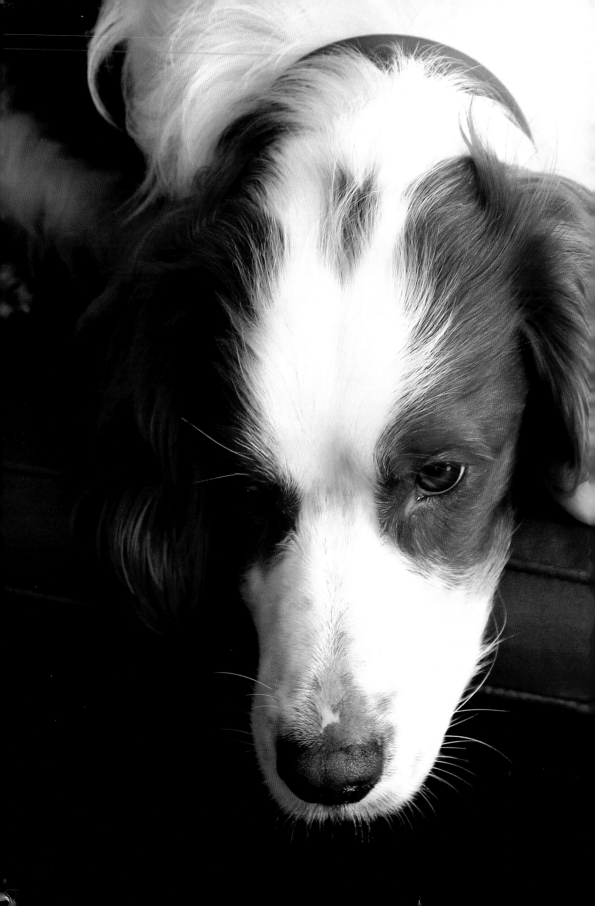

ROBERT FALCONER-TAYLOR
PETER NEVILLE
VAL STRONG

EMRA™
Intelligence

The EMRA™ Approach to
Pet Behaviour Problem Assessment
and Treatment

SitzPlatzFuss
edition

Copyright © 2014 Cadmos Publishing Limited, Richmond, UK
Copyright of original edition © 2013 Cadmos Verlag GmbH, Schwarzenbek, Germany
Design: Ravenstein + Partner, Verden
Setting: jb:design – Johanna Böhm, Dassendorf
Cover photograph: Tierfotoagentur
Content photos: Tierfotoagentur, unless otherwise indicated
Drawings: COAPE Institute
Editorial of original edition: Madeleine Franck
Editorial of this edition: Christopher Long
Printed by: Westermann Druck, Zwickau

British Library Cataloguing in Publication Data
A catalogue record of this book is available from the British Library.

Printed in Germany

ISBN: 978-0-85788-016-1

Contents

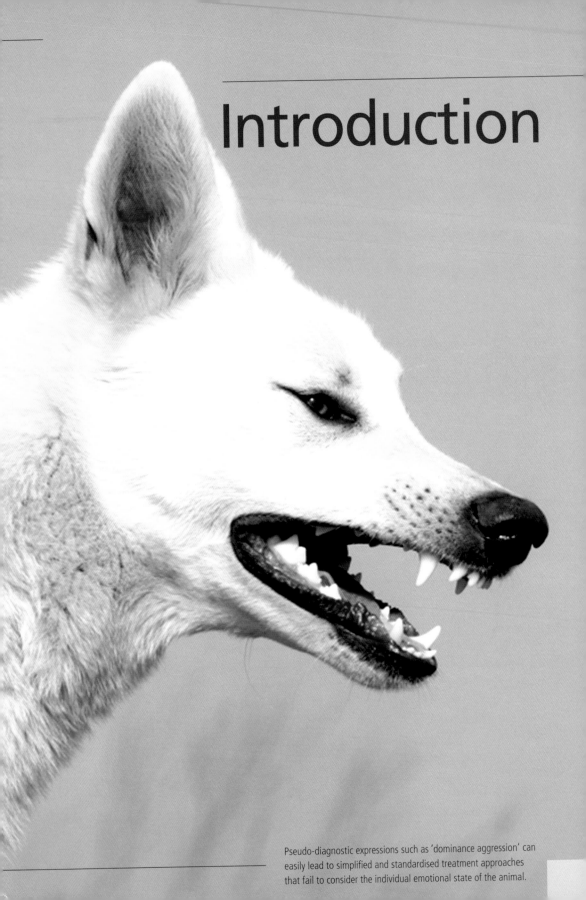

Introduction

Pseudo-diagnostic expressions such as 'dominance aggression' can easily lead to simplified and standardised treatment approaches that fail to consider the individual emotional state of the animal.

A fundamental, initially controversial, yet highly sensible change in the approach to the assessment and treatment of behaviour problems in companion animals has been established over the past few years at the Centre of Applied Pet Ethology (COAPE) in the UK. This has involved a major rethink of the global pseudo-diagnostic labelling techniques of old, such as 'dominance aggression' and 'separation anxiety'. These descriptions have been widely adopted over the years, because they are often very simple to grasp; however, as anyone in the street could doubtless testify, behaviour, normal or abnormal, problematic or acceptable, is rarely a simple subject!

The old-fashioned labels given to behaviour problems, and the accompanying attempts to classify them on the basis of those labels, have inspired standardised treatment approaches in behaviour therapy, used by many behaviourists and veterinary practices alike, and the increasingly automatic prescription of medication for behaviour cases by veterinary surgeons who find themselves trying to address problems within the short time constraints of a routine practice consultation. The rigid and unthinking application of these approaches, which are largely based on the practice of collecting 'sufficient and necessary' signs to conclude a 'diagnosis' of a behaviour problem, have ensured that behaviour problems in dogs and cats have become increasingly seen as arising from some clinical abnormality, i.e. it is assumed that companion animals with behaviour problems are pathologically abnormal. Yet the vast majority of animals presenting with behaviour problems are clinically healthy. Behaviour problems are not diseases, even if they can mimic the signs and symptoms of some clinical conditions. These standardised approaches often lead to the assumption that treatment requires the lifelong prescription of drugs to restrain the animals emotionally, and to provide permanent behavioural management so that the owners can have a hope of living with their pets happily and safely.

The result of all of this has been that many experienced and inexperienced behaviourists have been striving to find clinical explanations for all behaviour problems, and have forgotten where the roots of companion animal behaviourism lie. It also seems to have been forgotten that dogs and cats are, for the most part, extraordinarily adaptable and well suited to life with people. In the search for some underlying disorder to explain, and in order to be able to categorise, behaviour problems, the fundamental nature of the vast majority of cases seems all too often to have been ignored. That vast majority of behaviour problems do not occur as a result of some clinically definable abnormality in the pet, but because these particular animals are experiencing difficulties in trying to cope with some aspect of their day-to-day lives, either with us or with conspecifics, and this deviates from the owners' view of how they should behave. In the very small number of cases where pets with behaviour problems are not clinically normal, they will usually present with other physical or general neurological/behavioural signs rather than context-specific behaviour problems. This is why it has long been the bedrock of behaviourists that behaviour cases are only treated on referral by veterinary surgeons who are qualified and legally entitled to make those genuine diagnoses and to judge an animal's clinical state before referring it for behaviour therapy.

We tutors and practitioners at COAPE have long resisted the temptation to look first for conveniently packaged 'diagnoses' for behavioural problems in the animals that we treat. While we retain a need for solid knowledge of the very new understanding of how and why animals do what they do at the physiological and neurotransmitter level in the brain, and take account of the latest

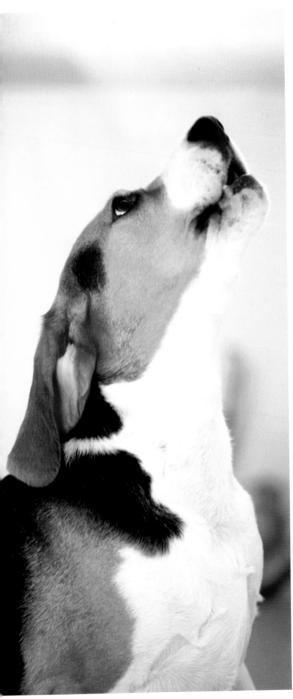

Dogs may howl or bark when they are left alone but this does not necessarily mean that they are suffering from 'separation anxiety'.

research publications on the genetic and experiential factors that influence behaviour, we remind ourselves constantly that the vast majority of companion animals with behaviour problems are clinically perfectly normal! The small number that are abnormal in no way justifies any need for behaviourists to become clinically expert at spotting them, because that is the job of the referring veterinary surgeon. Of course, with experience and help from veterinary surgeons well versed in genuine clinically abnormal cases, many behaviourists do become quite good at knowing what signs may contribute to a medically induced behavioural condition rather than a straightforward learned problem behaviour. These animals need patient and expert help so they can learn to behave differently, and usually in rather specific circumstances (e.g. Walker et al., 1997). They do not need a false, jargonised, quasi-scientific clinical diagnosis, an automated prescription of drugs, or standardised behaviour 'therapy' advice to help them get better at coping.

So if, as COAPE believes, one should resist the overly simplistic behavioural approaches of old, and if one refuses to adopt the idea that companion animals with behaviour problems are clinically abnormal, what then should one believe in? It is actually very simple. At COAPE we have developed, applied, teach and now widely propose a more sensitive and individual approach to each problem behaviour case, based on EMRA™ – the three tenets of:

1. *Emotional Assessment* of the animal at the time the problem is observed,
2. *Mood State Assessment* of how the animal feels and behaves generally, and
3. *Reinforcement Assessment* of exactly which factors, external and internal, are maintaining the behaviour problem, often in spite of many varied attempts to remove it.

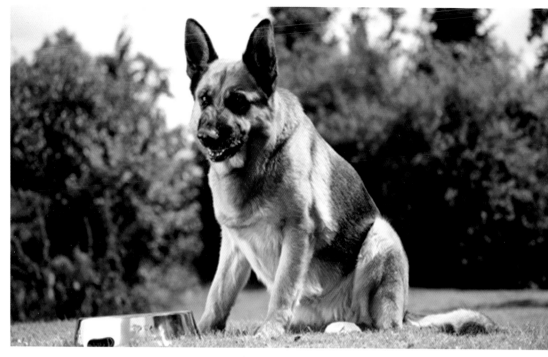

Food guarding may be a problem behaviour for the owner, but not for the dog!

At the core of this new approach lies an increased awareness of the *individuality* and *emotionality* of the animal, and the development of the practitioner's ability to interpret how it feels. This is a dangerously controversial and anthropomorphic concept for some, in the absence of scientific techniques to quantify emotionality, but it is a logical development, given the essential highly emotional nature of all mammals. This, in fact, forms the 'art' of being a good empathetic behavioural practitioner, as opposed to one who lectures his or her clients about what their animals have 'got', uses complex terminology to describe simple things and offers standardised approaches to treatment.

This 'art' is now based on hard science. The physical and physiological relationships between the structures of the brain that govern moments of fear and anger, pleasure and ecstasy have for some years been a subject of great activity in neurobiological research in the field of human psychiatry. For example, 'for many, emotional intelligence, ancient, impulsive and highly influential, determines our hopes for success as a species compared with our newer, more easily measured, cognitive intelligence, with its greater awareness and ability to ponder and reflect, and power to over-ride instinctive emotional responses' (Goleman, 1996). Others suggest that the interplay between the two seats of intelligence is fundamental, and our ability to be sensitive to our emotions but to govern them with cognitive analysis holds the key. However, the structure of the human brain seems to allow emotionally driven instinctive responses to override cognitive processes and controlled responses very naturally at certain times. When decisions and action are required, 'feeling counts every bit as much and, sometimes, more than thought. Intelligence can come to nothing when emotions hold sway', as one highly respected neurobiologist wrote (Le Doux, 1998).

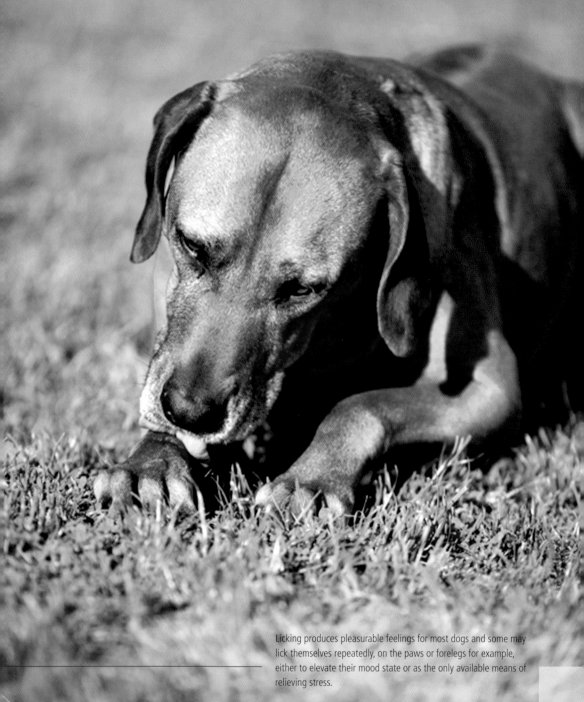

What are
Emotions?

Licking produces pleasurable feelings for most dogs and some may lick themselves repeatedly, on the paws or forelegs for example, either to elevate their mood state or as the only available means of relieving stress.

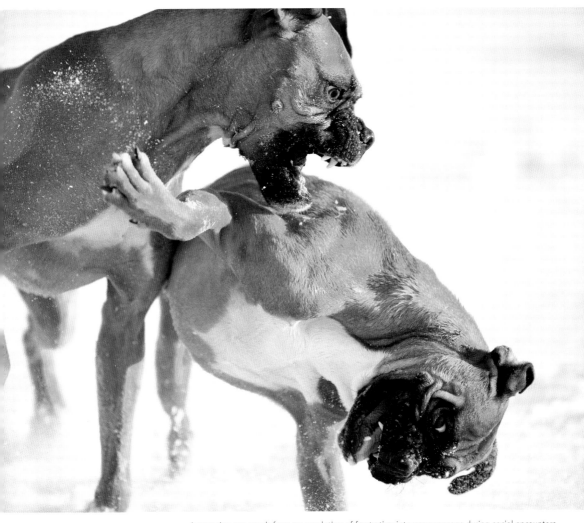

Aggression can result from an escalation of frustration into anger or rage during social encounters, or from excitement that is misinterpreted by the other dog as threatening behaviour.

Emotions can be described as impulses to act, and as states of mind produced by reinforcing stimuli for very specific purposes. These include arousing the animal to take action to defend itself, seek food or other necessities, to form and maintain cooperative attachments with others in a group (for obligatory social animals such as dogs), to communicate emotional states one to another, to respond to novelty, and to memorise signals and happenings associated with social or environmental events and to learn to respond to those signals in the future, particularly in the case of stimuli associated with danger. Indeed, the different emotions may be classified according to whether the reinforcer is positive or negative. This gives rise to scales of reinforcement contingencies related to degrees of emotionality, e.g. pleasure increasing to elation and ecstasy, frustration increasing to anger and rage, apprehension increasing to fear and terror, etc. (see Figure 1, after Rolls, 1999).

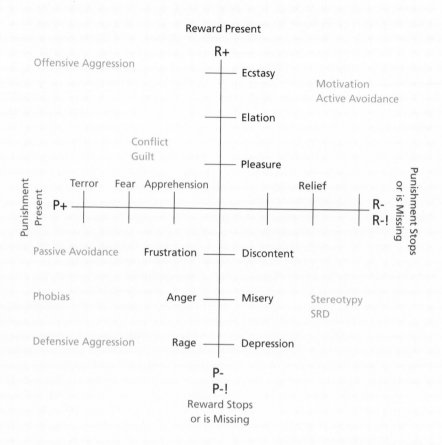

Figure 1:

1. External triggers influence the emotional state – if the dog has an extrovert character and is able to react actively, frustration may develop into ANGER/RAGE, but if the dog is more introverted and/or can only react passively, it may develop into MISERY/DEPRESSION.

2. Feelings can be complicated mixtures of emotions. A good example in people might be the CONFLICT/GUILT/PLEASURE experienced during an extramarital affair or FEAR/JOY/RELIEF during a bungee jump.

3. RELIEF is a very powerful and sometimes overwhelming emotion, and experiencing relief can develop into an addiction. For example in the pursuit of high-risk sports, such as parachuting, a person repeatedly exposes themselves to a fear-inducing situation in order to experience the great feelings of relief at surviving a successful jump.

4. An intense feeling of pleasure is highly rewarding and can also lead to addictive behaviour, which is the main reason behind drug abuse.

5. To be able to interpret and understand emotions it is vital to pay careful attention to body language, facial expressions, and the speed and relative direction of movement.

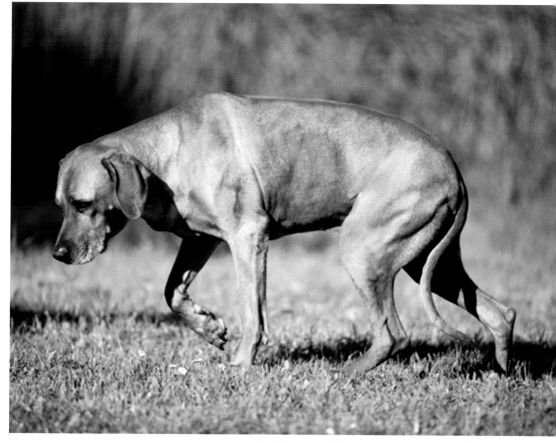

To be able to understand and change a dog's behaviour it is essential to assess their emotional state. Being able to read the dog's body language is a vital part of this assessment.

When working with the EMRA™ model, making an Emotional Assessment of a dog that is behaving aggressively towards another, or a dog that is destructive when left at home alone, is a vital first step. This is not a diagnosis, because only veterinary and medical practitioners are legally allowed to make diagnoses. This may be seen as commercial self-protection by some, and may fuel a need to classify all behaviour problems as if they are clinical diseases, or abnormalities lying solely within the animal. Rather than seeking to diagnose, it is essential to form an opinion of how the dog actually feels at the time of the problem: to assess whether it is fearful, frustrated, angry, sad,

happy, etc. All of these emotions differ, and an accurate assessment points the way to treatment. The focus of treatment is first to decide how would we like the dog to feel as an alternative in such circumstances. We would obviously like to help a fearful dog to feel more confident or an angry dog to feel more content, and the job of the behaviourist is to help them learn to get there.

Making a Mood State Assessment of how the dog feels and behaves generally, at all other times when not showing the problem behavior, is our next step. Clearly a depressed dog is much harder to motivate in treatment than a more content one, but a maniacally happy dog that loves everyone

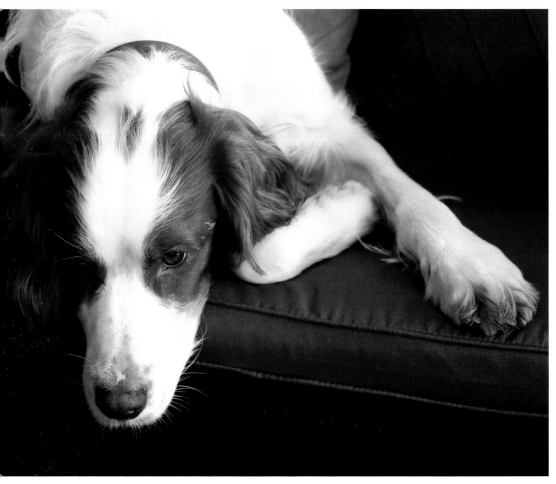

A dog's mood state needs to be relaxed and positive before any changes to their emotional state and resulting behaviour in the problem situation can be addressed.

and everything is in just as difficult a mood if, for example, we want them to focus and learn how to be calm with another dog instead of leaping all over them and frightening them. (Boxer owners will recognise this – their dogs get into trouble sometimes and then become aggressive because they are just too exuberant for other dogs!) It is the dog's basal mood state that first needs attention, not their emotional response at the time that they get into conflict with other dogs. That comes after we have stabilised mood at a more relaxed and communicable level.

The third part of the EMRA™ approach is Reinforcement Assessment, which involves assessing what the benefit is to the dog in actually performing the problem behaviour. If there were no emotional benefit to the dog, the behaviour would never have been established or repeated, or withstood any efforts to remove it. This is crucial, as the question of reinforcement must also be considered at the neurochemical level, and any treatment must first uncouple the feelings of success or relief that have become established when carrying out the behaviour. Only then can one develop opportunities in treatment for the dog to carry out alternative, but equally successful or relief-bringing, behaviours which themselves become reinforced and established in those circumstances.

Learning produces changes in the way animals perceive their physical and social environment, and also the way they feel emotionally in their responses to signals associated with dangers or rewards. For example, it is no easier to separate emotionality from the complexities of learning and maintaining social behaviour than it is from obviously rewarding events, such as responses to signals associated with the discovery of food, which have been traditionally described as rather unemotional 'conditioned' responses (e.g. in Pavlov's classic conditioning experiments with dogs). The purpose of emotions in these instances is to equip the body to 'do something' about events in the environment, and the signals associated with them, and to shape, intensify, refine and perfect the behaviours that gain rewards. This is especially so with the primary rewards of food, sex, social contact and safety, even though the associated behaviours are naturally innately reinforcing in themselves. In fact, the reason why mammals are so successful is that they are so emotionally sensitive, and have the capability to assess the 'value' of every sensory input very rapidly indeed; i.e. is it good/bad or neutral to their wellbeing? It is also true to say that, whether one considers newly acquired learning in novel situations, or the refinement of the expressions of inbuilt heritable motor patterns of behaviour, *there is no learning without emotional change*. Ultimately a positive emotional change at the neurophysiological level, for example from fear to relief or from neutral to happiness, is the reinforcement for any behaviour.

It is therefore a mistake automatically to label the animal that grooms and licks itself to the point of mutilation as suffering from a clinical 'obsessive–compulsive disorder' (OCD), despite the urge to reach for a complex description for such a seemingly bizarre behaviour. It may in fact be the response of a perfectly normal dog or cat that is under considerable stress, for example as a result of being socially isolated or denied opportunity to fulfil normal mood-sustaining behaviours. Denied features that are important to the maintenance of its normal species- or type-specific mood state balance, a dog may carry out the only available behaviour that induces positive emotional changes, to try and maintain its mood. One behaviour that makes a dog, or indeed a person, feel better is self-grooming. For some dogs, a little chewing of toys brings relief, for others a lot of chewing, perhaps of themselves, is the only option available. Restore the general mood of the dog by providing opportunities to perform other innately rewarding behaviours, and the dog is better equipped to cope with emotional upheaval without relying on the outlet of licking or chewing itself like a comfort blanket. It is all so logical – there is no need to classify an 'OCD' clinically as if the licking or chewing is a disease. There is also no need in many cases to medicate the animal, especially if treatment occurs before the behaviour becomes addictive, i.e. performed for its emotional benefits at times when the dog is not isolated or otherwise stressed.

Equally, it is rather pointless to offer a range of behaviour treatments to improve the dog's mood state if no account is taken of the highly variable specific behavioural needs of the type of dog presented. Jack Russell Terriers clearly have different requirements from German Shepherd Dogs, Border Collies or Pyrenean Mountain Dogs for maintaining their normal mood state, and these, along with factors such as age, sex and individual personality, must be individually addressed in each case (COAPE, 2012).

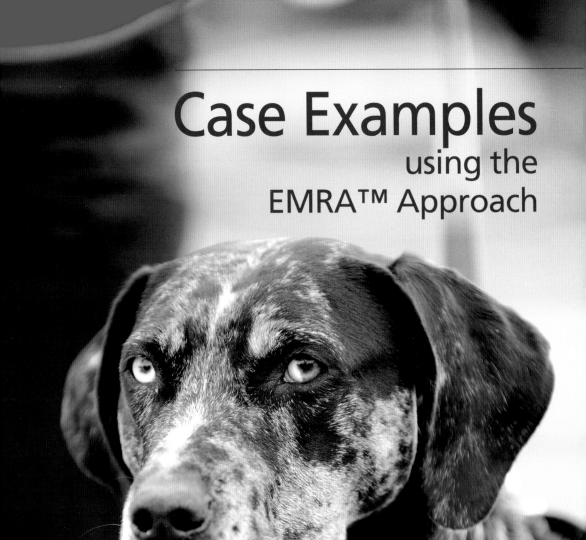

Case Examples
using the
EMRA™ Approach

The following seven case histories present various real-life cases
treated by different authors, all of whom are either Partners/Tutors
in COAPE, or holders of the COAPE Diploma in Companion Animal
Behaviour Therapy and Training (DipCABT), which has been taught
by COAPE in the UK since 1997. All authors are members of the
COAPE Association of Pet Behaviourists and Trainers
(see www.capbt.org). The style and language of presentation
varies slightly in the seven cases because the EMRA™ approach
is specifically designed to encourage each COAPE behaviour
practitioner to develop their own evidence-based, yet vitally
empathetic, assessment and treatment style.

CASE HISTORY 1:
Fear of Strangers

DOGS:
Ben, German Shepherd Dog;
Max, Labrador Retriever
AGE:
Ben: 3 years approx; Max: 18 months
DEX:
Ben: Male; Max: Male (neutered)
PROBLEM:
Both dogs are fearful of strangers

When attempting to modify an animal's behaviour, it is important to consider and try to understand the surge of feelings (emotions) the animal is experiencing during the unwanted behaviour and also its baseline, or average, feelings (mood state) during the rest of the day. A human example might help to explain why.

Imagine your 10-year-old son is playing football outside the kitchen window and you have already asked him, to no avail, to go and play in the garden so as not to kick the ball through the window. A while later, the ball smashes through the kitchen window. Your initial emotion might be one of anger at your son for not doing as he was asked. Now consider the same scenario, but this time you have flu with a grumbling headache and feel irritable. The ball comes crashing though the kitchen window. What is your emotional response to the event this time? Explosive anger, probably. Or maybe resignation because you are too tired or exasperated to bother.

Everyone has their own particular general mood state that fluctuates in every direction by a small amount around some average throughout the day. A person suffering from depression will have a very different mood state from someone who is happy and contented with life, and these two people will have a very different emotional reaction to the same event. These feelings can be mixed; for example, a person making a parachute jump for the first time might feel pleasure, even elation, along with apprehension or fear.

Emotional Assessment

The beauty of the EMRA™ model is that both the type of emotion experienced during a problem behaviour and its intensity can be represented diagrammatically. This is extremely useful for both the behaviour practitioner *and* the animal's owner when trying to unravel and interpret what is going on (COAPE, 2012). For example, there may be several reasons why a dog barks at strangers when out walking with their owner in the park (see Figure 2). Ben, a German Shepherd Dog, is

Failing to develop effective communication can dramatically affect a dog's general mood state. This can cause or exacerbate many behaviour problems because of the resulting anxiety and lack of predictability of the owner's intentions for the dog.

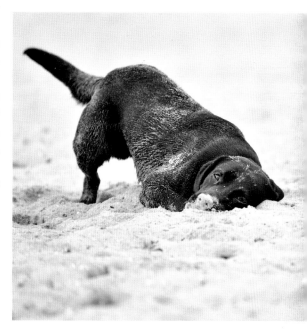

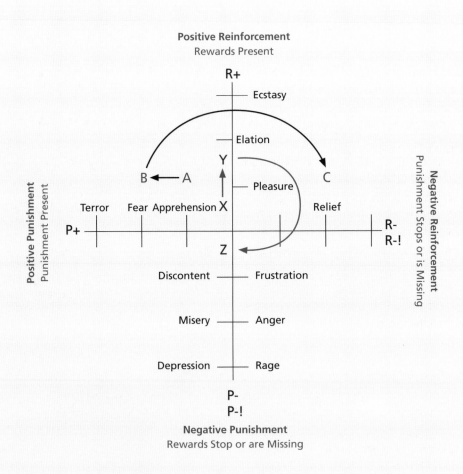

Figure 2: Assessment of the emotional states shown by Ben and Max

fearful of strangers and has learned that barking at them causes them to retreat, or his owner to walk him quickly in another direction. Either way, the result for Ben is that his fear changes to a feeling of relief as the distance between him and the stranger is increased. In such a case, when Ben first spots the stranger at a distance, his first emotion may be apprehension (point A, Figure 2), but then as the stranger approaches, Ben will become fearful (point B) and start to bark to try and halt the stranger's advance. If the threat is successful, Ben's fear declines and he experiences the emotion of relief (point C) as the stranger recedes.

Max is an entire 18-month-old Labrador Retriever, and he also barks at strangers. Max, however, barks because he has learned that it attracts attention from his owner, even if this is negative attention in the form of being told off. In this case, Max might first feel pleasure (moving from point X to point Y, Figure 2) from his owner's attention, which then turns into frustration (point Z) as he is pulled in the opposite direction and away from the stranger.

Mood State Assessment

The physiological homoeostasis of blood glucose levels, body temperature, hunger, thirst, heart rate and so on is well understood. What is less well recognised is that mood state is also subject to homoeostatic regulation. In the same way as other homoeostatic mechanisms maintain physiological equilibrium within the body, the emotional brain maintains an individual's so-called Hedonic Set Point (HSP), tending to pull any emotional divergence back to its 'normal' level (Koob and Le Moal, 1997; COAPE, 2012).

Figure 3 illustrates the relationship between mood state and the HSP. The point of Resting

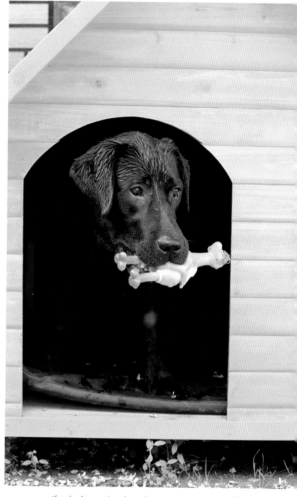

If a dog's emotional needs are not being met sufficiently they may search for opportunities to maintain and improve their general mood for themselves.

Contentment, running through the centre of the diagram, is the pivotal point around which fluctuations in mood occur; 'good feelings' are above the line and 'bad feelings' below. Resting Contentment is defined as having no particular feelings at all, such as just before falling asleep. If you imagine an animal's mood state being attached to the line of Resting Contentment by elastic bands, any changes in mood in either direction (positive or negative) will tend to be pulled back

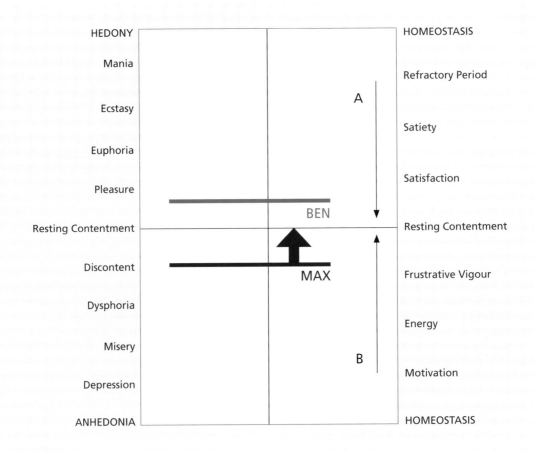

Figure 3: Assessment of the mood states of Ben and Max

towards the centre (lines A and B, Figure 3). In a normal, contented animal the HSP lies somewhere just above the line of Resting Contentment and represents feelings of satisfaction and wellbeing. In order to maintain the HSP, this animal will actively pursue normal, everyday behaviours that are both rewarding and pleasurable *to them*.

Going back to the example of the dogs that bark at people in the park, Figure 3 shows diagrammatically the Mood State Assessment for Ben and Max. Ben is an only dog and has love and attention lavished upon him in abundance by his owners in the form of inventive training and games. His mood state, we would suggest, is where it should be; somewhere just above the point of Resting Contentment.

In contrast, Max, the entire 18-month-old Labrador, lives with a couple who have just had a new baby and consequently he no longer enjoys as many walks or as much attention. He has become more boisterous and is no longer let off the lead when out on a walk. Recently, he has started to guard objects such as socks and shoes and he growls at his owners when they try to retrieve them. When confronted with a dog like Max in the consulting room, how many behaviourists and veterinarians would recommend that he should be neutered as their first line of treatment? Yet where would you estimate Max's mood state to be? Can you see why, from the information provided, we would place it below the line in Figure 3? In this example, Max's mood state is likely to be pushed down, because his emotional needs are no longer being met, and his behaviour is driven by his frustration to 'push' his mood state back up again. This helps to explain why castrating Max is unlikely to have any positive effect on his behaviour.

Reinforcement Assessment

Consideration of the emotional needs of an individual, of any species, is not the fanciful brainchild of some ambitious social worker. Different types of dog (e.g. hounds, gundogs, terriers, sighthounds and toy dogs) are good at doing different things. This may seem a rather obvious statement, but it lies at the heart of many frustratingly persistent behaviour problems in dogs. To understand why, we need to take a fresh look at the wolf as the dog's original ancestor and, in particular, the wolf's predatory behaviour.

Like all predatory animals, the wolf has a genetically inherited motor pattern of behaviour called the 'predatory sequence', which is hard-wired into its brain. This pattern is triggered by the sight of a prey animal, and directs the hungry wolf through a predetermined sequence of behaviours that ultimately ends in a meal, provided all goes according to plan (see Figure 4a). It is important to realise that it is this predatory sequence that makes it impossible to domesticate the wolf. A wolf brought up with human beings is indeed tame – and very dangerous – because if someone inadvertently triggers the predatory sequence, that person would most likely end up as lunch. The domestic dog is genetically almost identical to the wolf, but the idea that the original domestic dog's ancestors were wolves captured and 'domesticated' by ancient humans has now been discredited (Coppinger and Coppinger, 2001).

Figure 4: Predatory motor pattern in wolves and dogs

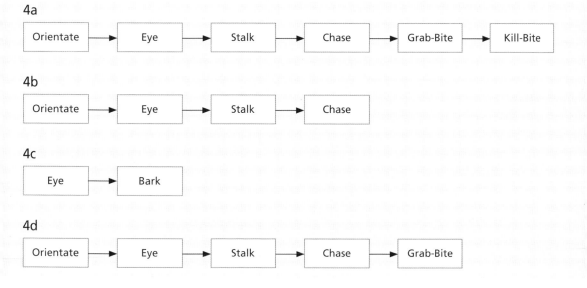

21

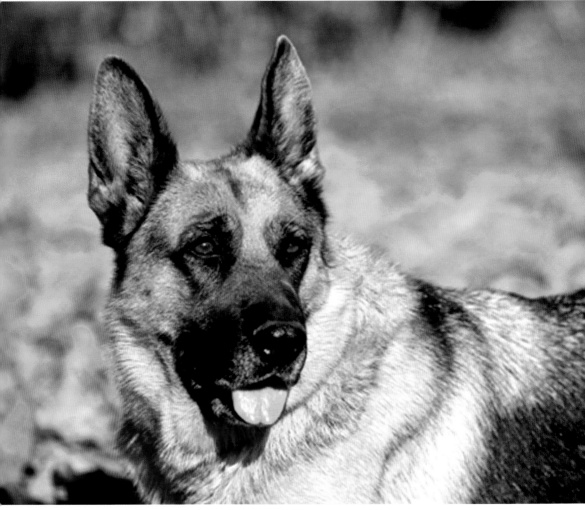

The emotional influences behind any particular behaviour problem may vary enormously among dogs.

The three survival imperatives for any animal are feeding, reproduction and staying out of trouble. Physical changes in an animal are triggered by changes in the environment and its behavioural adaptations to ensure survival. The change in the environment that facilitated the domestication of the wolf into the dog occurred 10,000 to 15,000 years ago, when humans began to adopt a village way of life. This provided the possibility of a year-round stable food supply for wild animals if they could move near enough to exploit it.

The rubbish dumps just outside villages and settlements would certainly have been a good source of 'scavengeable' food for some wolves and many other animals who could tolerate the relatively close proximity of humans. The dumps would also have provided a safe place for juvenile wolves to be left by the adults when they went on hunting excursions. Although past the very dependent cub stage and out of the den, these juveniles would not yet be old or experienced enough with their hunting and communication skills to join the hunt for wild quarry, but would need to be left in a safe place. Dumps would be ideal as they contained small 'snack' prey such as rodents, and edible waste left by humans, which would help the young wolves survive if the pack returned late or not at all. Other predators that might prey on young wolves, such as large cats, are mainly solitary and more sensitive to disturbance and would have been less likely to approach human settlements.

The wolves that benefited most from this stable food supply and security of the out-of-town dumps were those that learned to live and survive close to humans without running away. The more confident juvenile wolves would soon have become able to follow people (seen as food-providing 'parent' figures) into the village to scavenge on the richer resources of the waste left in the streets and on the contents of village latrines, which provided food for vermin and canine scavengers alike. All of this biodegradable waste was of no use to the humans in the villages, but it could be utilised by dogs and converted into canine protein for humans to eat. So, while it was probably the case that humans could not have chased the young wolves away even if they had wanted to, there was an ulterior motive to want them around. The switch from a hunter/gatherer lifestyle to mainly crop farming would have meant that an easily obtainable year-round meat supply would have been highly advantageous. Young wolves would have provided this buffer to poor harvests and so it would have suited humans to tolerate their scavenging activities in the villages. Once a resident population of young wolves was established in the village and had stayed to reach maturity and breed there, the people would soon have become aware of which wolf/dogs produced the biggest, fastest-growing puppies and encouraged them to stay to provide food later. Direct physical contact and socialisation of village-born puppies with humans would then have

occurred as a crucial part of the taming and domestication process.

Early village dogs would therefore have been indirectly encouraged to grow up while retaining the playful characteristics of juvenile wolves, and not to develop the organised social or predatory behaviours typical of adult wolves, in order for humans to accept them without danger to themselves. These juvenile characteristics thus became established in the adult, reproductive population of village dogs. Some would have retained near-adult qualities in terms of their predatory behaviour patterns, and they would have been ideal for helping people to stalk prey when they went out to hunt. Similarly, such dogs could also have proved useful in helping to herd sheep and other livestock outside the village, but only once the bite/kill end of the hunting sequence had been selected out (Figure 4b) by culling any dogs that attacked livestock, or using them instead for hunting. Village dogs that remained very juvenile in their behaviour and showed no propensity to hunt or herd would have been ideal for guarding livestock (Figure 4c). Other slightly more adult types would have developed possessive instincts and these would have been selected and trained to use as retrievers on the hunt (Figure 4d). Thus herding, stalking, heeling, retrieving and guarding types of dog would all have evolved in the early villages from less socially competitive, less predatory animals.

Thus, the different *types* of dog around today may be classified according to the fragments of their wolf ancestors' predatory motor patterns they have retained and how much these fragments have been hypertrophied, suppressed or otherwise altered by natural selection, or deliberately by humans. In certain breeds of dog the motivation to perform specialised routines such as retrieving or herding may be so intense that frustration ensues when no opportunities for work

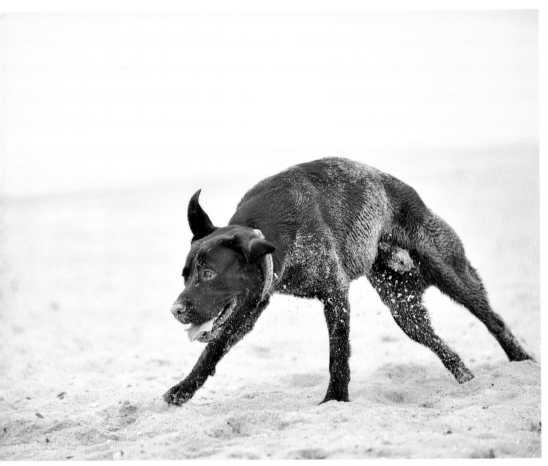

The reward for any behaviour is ultimately based on a positive emotional change at the neurophysiological level. If it makes you feel good, you will learn and repeat the behaviour that earned the reward!

or appropriate play alternatives exist. This situation will be made very much worse by punishment of the behaviour in question. Clear instances abound where retrievers have been taught to become aggressive by repeated punishment of their innocent compulsions to retrieve anything and everything. Some very severe attacks upon owners by their dogs can be explained fully in this way, for example in some cases of so-called 'rage syndrome' in Cocker Spaniels and Golden Retrievers (see later).

Back to Ben and Max: On the surface, their behaviour, barking at people in the park, would appear to be the same; however, the emotions involved are very different, as clearly illustrated by their respective Emotional Assessments (Figure 2). This gives us some clues about where to look when making the Reinforcement Assessment for each dog. Both dogs are being rewarded by their behaviour (if they were not, then the behaviour would have ceased on its own). The obvious reward for Ben is that barking 'makes' the stranger recede. In addition, Ben's Emotional Assessment tells us that he experiences relief as a result, an emotional change from fear that is a very powerful reinforcer indeed to the behaviour he employs to make that happen. Finally, the way Ben's owner reacts to him, by instinctively jerking back on the lead, contains yet another 'hidden' reward for the behaviour, reinforcing it even more (this is Mowrer's Two-Factor Theory – for a dog-specific reference, see Lindsay, 2000). *All* of these reinforcers have to be identified and systematically removed if Ben's behaviour problem is going to be satisfactorily resolved.

Another equally important part of the Reinforcement Assessment is the consideration of what rewarding activities can be utilised in a behaviour modification programme. In order to change an undesirable behaviour it is not enough simply to stop the animal from performing that behaviour; rather, the animal needs to be taught some alternative behaviour that is *equally or even more rewarding*. It could be that the undesirable behaviour has arisen because, being denied the opportunity to perform some important inbuilt behavioural motor pattern, the animal has resorted to doing something else in an attempt to maintain their HSP. For Max, this is precisely the problem. From his Emotional Assessment (Figure 2) and Mood State Assessment (Figure 3), it is clear that the driving force behind his behaviour is essentially emotional deprivation and no amount of 'behaviour modification' is going to address his problems.

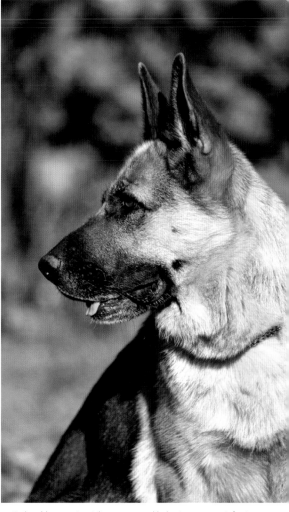

To be able to extinguish an unwanted behaviour every reinforcing factor needs to be identified and consistently removed.

The Brain Reward System and the Concept of Therapy-induced Frustration

The neurotransmitters, located in the limbic system, responsible for the Brain Reward System's (BRS) feelings of pleasure, reward and wellbeing have collectively been called the Reward Cascade (Blum et al., 1996).

'*The cascade begins with the excitatory activity of serotonin-releasing neurons in the hypothala-mus. This causes the release of the opioid peptide met-encephalin in the ventral tegmental area, which inhibits the activity of neurons that release the inhibitory neurotransmitter gamma-aminobutyric acid (GABA). The disinhibition of dopamine-containing neurons in the ventral tegmental area allows them to release dopamine in the nucleus accumbens and in certain parts of the hippocampus, permitting the completion of the cascade.*'

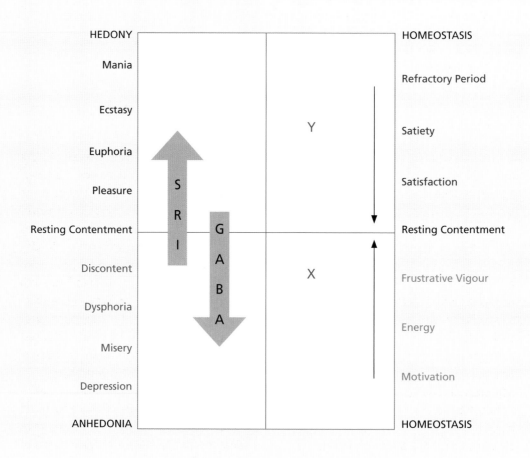

Figure 5: Effects of GABA and SRIs.

A disruption anywhere in this finely balanced chain of excitatory and inhibitory reactions can result in anxiety, anger and other 'bad feelings', or an extreme behaviour that alleviates the negative emotion. For a comprehensive review of the BRS, see Naranjo *et al.* (2001).

COAPE (2012) raises the intriguing possibility of therapy-induced frustration and the use of 'pharmacological probes'. The Reward Cascade theory of Blum and others (1996) predicts that GABA agonists (e.g. barbiturates, benzodiazepines) will tend to reduce the degree of reward an animal derives from a given activity. Conversely, serotonin agonists (e.g. serotonin reuptake inhibitors (SRIs), such as clomipramine) will tend to increase the degree of reward an animal derives from a given activity.

Thus, the influence that such drugs are likely to have on an animal's behaviour depends on the level at which its mood state resides at the time. For example, point X in Figure 5 shows an animal with a depressed mood state, where there will be a tendency (frustrative vigour) for it to adopt behaviours that elevate its mood state. In such an animal, barbiturates would tend to increase frustrative vigour as the animal has to work even harder to push its mood state upwards, and so the behaviour worsens. SRIs would tend to have the opposite effect, helping to re-establish hedonic homoeostasis with an improvement in the behaviour. Conversely, for an animal with an already elevated mood state at point Y in Figure 5, the exact opposite would tend to occur.

Mills (2003) rightly cautions against attempting to make a diagnosis of a psychological disorder on the basis of a patient's response to a particular drug. However, the use of BRS agonists and antagonists as pharmacological probes has, in our experience, proved useful in helping to unravel the Emotional Assessment and Mood State Assessment for some more complex behavioural cases.

CASE HISTORY 2:
Over-excitement, nipping and clothes-tearing

DOG:
Sam, Labrador Retriever
AGE:
9 months
SEX:
Male (neutered)
PROBLEM:
Over-excitement, nipping and clothes-tearing

This case is described and then analysed using the COAPE (2012) EMRA™ model. A standard behavioural workup was carried out which included a detailed question and answer session, and passive observation of the dog's behaviour and interactions with the owners both indoors and outdoors. In addition, the owners were requested to obtain video footage that represented a typical day at home with their dog including, if possible, footage of the problem behaviours if this did not put anyone at risk of being injured. The dog underwent a complete physical examination and haematology and biochemistry screening, and no abnormalities were found.

The owners were advised on the basics of training, including the importance of rewarding correct behaviour and not inadvertently rewarding (reinforcing) incorrect behaviour. In the interests of brevity, details of the client training and behaviour modification plans are not discussed here.

Sam presented with a long-standing problem of excitability and lack of control, problems which had recently developed into more overt aggressive challenges towards the owners, leading them to seek professional help. The owners were a retired couple and had owned many dogs in the past, including Labradors. They had acquired this

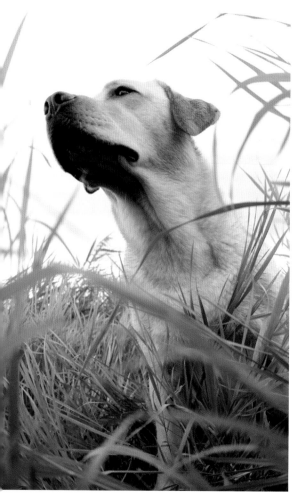

The perfect dog in class, but misbehaving at home! A dog that is out of control and excitable at home shows all too clearly that something is amiss in his everyday life irrespective of how well he focuses and learns at training classes.

trainees. He was taken for one or two walks per day of an hour or more. The owners described his behaviour as variable from one walk to the next but generally worse when Mr X was present. One day he could be a pleasure to take out with good recall, playing with his ball and with other dogs, whereas on other occasions Sam pulled on the lead and jumped up, pulling at clothing, had no interest in his ball and ran off ignoring the owners when called.

At home the problem behaviour was directed primarily at Mr X. Whenever he walked into the house Sam jumped up and pulled at his clothing (several garments had been destroyed) and mouthed his hands and wrists – up until recently the skin was not usually punctured. The same behaviour occurred following walks when Mr X tried to remove his jacket. This behaviour also occurred at other times, such as when Mr X was sitting reading the newspaper, watching television, or when he raised his voice. At times the dog settled comfortably at his owners' feet in the lounge, whereas at other times he retired on his own to his basket upstairs for several hours at a time during the day. At other times he did not settle, running from one end of the house to the other, jumping on the furniture, nipping the owners as he passed by, barking and chewing up anything he found. This sometimes happened late at night after the owners had gone to bed. To date, Sam had damaged fitted carpets, kitchen floor lino and furniture. He also exhibited tail-chasing behaviour that was becoming more prolonged in duration and frequency.

Interventions that had been tried by the owners prior to consultation included: (a) time out by shutting Sam in the bathroom, (b) pulling him down by the collar and pinning him to the floor, (c) seizing him in a bear-hug around his abdomen, (d) smacking. Of these, only (a) and (c) were helpful.

particular dog at 8 weeks of age and, according to them, 'he had always been a handful'.

Sam was well socialised with other dogs and with people including children. His diet consisted of a top brand complete life stage mix and an assortment of small treats. He attended weekly training classes and was described by the trainer as 'the model dog'; the trainer often used him to demonstrate what she wanted from the other

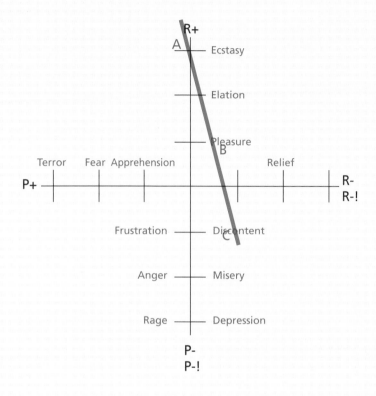

Figure 6: Assessment of Sam's emotional state.

Emotional Assessment

An Emotional Assessment for the case is shown in Figure 6. While engaged in the undesirable behaviour Sam's emotional state fluctuated considerably around the pivotal point B, the driving force of discontent and frustration. As time went on, the behaviour became more extreme, sometimes peaking in pleasure (point A) and at other times troughing in anger and displays of aggres-

sion (point C). The key point to remember here is that an individual's emotions are fluid and can switch very rapidly from one state to another.

Mood State Assessment

Our Mood State Assessment for the case is shown in Figure 7. Sam's mood state was depressed (point B) and his behaviour was directed at trying

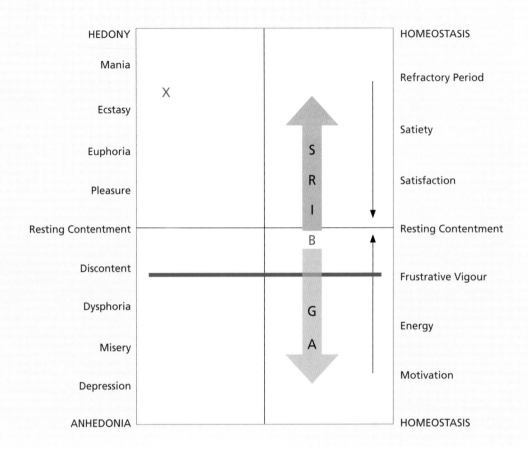

HEDONY

Mania

Ecstasy

Euphoria

Pleasure

Resting Contentment

Discontent

Dysphoria

Misery

Depression

ANHEDONIA

HOMEOSTASIS

Refractory Period

Satiety

Satisfaction

Resting Contentment

Frustrative Vigour

Energy

Motivation

HOMEOSTASIS

Figure 7: Assessment of Sam's mood state.

to elevate it. The owners, however, were adamant that their dog had a 'clinical abnormality' and were not convinced that the behaviour was driven by frustration (see Bowen (2002) for a discussion on overactivity vs. hyperactivity/hyperkinesis), and at this point were considering euthanasia. The possibility of being able to 'test' Sam (see the discussion on therapy-induced frustration above) was therefore offered as a way forward and, with the owners' informed consent, the dog was administered phenobarbitone. Within a few days, the owners reported back that Sam's behaviour had become dramatically worse. The phenobarbitone was withdrawn and clomipramine prescribed. The owners reported an overall improvement in behaviour, which was maintained as long as the dog remained on the drug. In our opinion, the phenobarbitone made the behaviour dramatically worse because it was exerting a 'downward pressure' on an already depressed mood state. Clomipramine, on the other hand, had the opposite effect because it was exerting an 'upward pressure' on Sam's mood state so that he could work a little less hard to satisfy his needs for rewards and pleasure. Had the dog's mood state been at point X in Figure 7, one would expect clomipramine to have made the behaviour worse and phenobarbitone to have improved it.

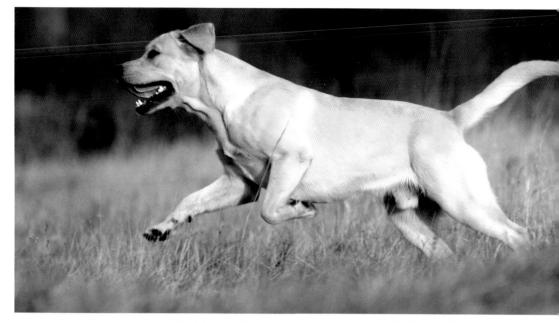

The Labrador retriever has a reputation for being the 'perfect family dog', but this can lead to misconceptions about the real emotional needs of this agile and potentially hardworking breed.

Reinforcement Assessment

Any owner who spends time observing their dog's daily 'habits' will gain a great deal of useful information about the dog's particular behavioural traits

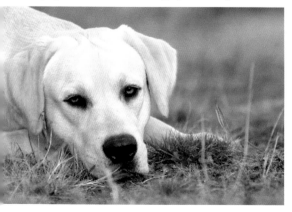

The EMRA™ system can help to determine whether more stimulation, mental challenges and activity might be useful, as with a relaxed but bored individual, or perhaps be counterproductive in a dog that gets easily agitated or aroused without appropriate training.

in relation to its original 'working type'. Here are some examples of common type-specific motor patterns.

- Retrievers – carrying or just holding objects in their mouths.
- Bassett Hounds – sniffing at the expense of any exercise, to the frustration of many owners.
- Border Collies – the *eye–stalk* part of the predatory sequence is extremely well developed, and these dogs experience a great deal of reward when engaged in this activity. In fact, some Border Collies become 'addicted' and will spend most of their waking hours eye–stalking anything that moves, at the expense of doing anything else. Imagine such a Border Collie that maintains his mood state by standing at a window all day watching passers-by on the street outside. The owners, in order to gain some privacy from the pedestrians looking back at the dog in amusement as they walk by, erect a high fence in front of the window,

31

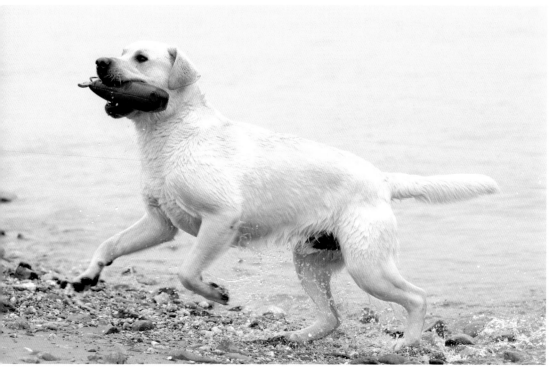

Retrievers experience carrying items in their mouths as highly and innately rewarding without additional external rewards from their owner, and so dummy work and retrieval games can be an excellent and easy way to improve their Hedonic Budgets.

thereby completely blocking the dog's view. Such a dog would inevitably undergo a mood state shift downwards towards frustration or even depression. He may then adopt other behaviours (e.g. chewing furniture, barking incessantly, snapping at his owners' heels as they walk around the house) in a desperate attempt to gain alternative rewards to drive his mood state back up again.

These behavioural sequences are hard-wired into the dog's brain and so performing them is innately rewarding and pleasurable, and may be very important for maintaining the dog's general mood state. Therefore, when dealing with a behavioural problem, the important question to ask is always:

'Which rewarding opportunities/activities that are important to the animal might be utilised in a behaviour modification programme, and which important opportunities/activities might be missing?'

These factors cannot be divorced from any treatment plan. In order to change an undesirable behaviour it is not enough simply to stop the animal from performing the behaviour. It is crucial that the animal learns for itself some alternative behaviour that is equally or even more rewarding. It could be that the undesirable behaviour has arisen because, being denied the opportunity to perform some important inbuilt behavioural motor pattern, the animal has resorted to doing something else in an attempt to maintain its mood.

It was concluded that there was nothing clinically wrong with Sam; he was just trying to be a Retriever. He responded well to training with chew and retrieval toys and thrived when given challenging exercises to do. Although the owners found Sam's behaviour acceptable when medicated with clomipramine, this was not offered as a solution. The recommendation was that Sam needed to be worked, but the owners were too elderly and frail to participate in an activity such as agility. Sam was therefore re-homed with a family that had two indoor pet Labradors that were recreationally worked at weekends. When followed up 6 months later the new owners reported that 'he was a wonderful dog both indoors and outdoors and they had experienced no problems with him whatsoever, and would not part with him for anything'. It is these authors' opinion that had this dog stayed with his original owners, he would have eventually been euthanased on the grounds of 'aggression'.

CASE HISTORY 3:
Soiling

DOG:
Mimi, Long-haired Miniature Dachshund
AGE:
3.5 years
SEX:
Female
PROBLEM:
Urinating on the owners'
bed at bedtime

This is an interesting case history where mood state dramatically influenced a specific behaviour problem, and attention to stabilising the dog's mood at a better level of 'resting contentment' provided the key to treatment, rather than focusing attention on the dog's emotionality or behaviour at the time the problem presented.

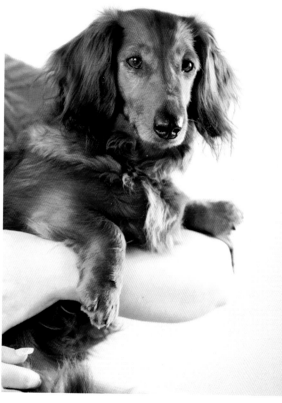

Dogs that are used to constant close physical contact with their owners are often very sensitive to their moods.

Being owned by a veterinarian and living in a house adjoining a large and well-equipped veterinary practice, the dog had already been regularly examined and no abnormalities were found. A standard behavioural workup was carried out, which included a detailed question and answer session and detailed personal observations of the dog's behaviour and interactions with the owners by Peter Neville, who was a guest in the house and practice for 5 days. (*See Photo 1: Peter Neville and Mimi.*)

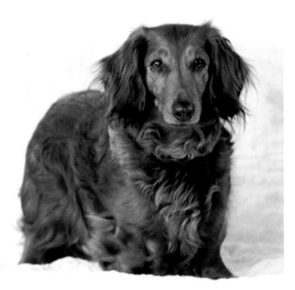

If it is important for a dog to sleep in their owner's bed an existing behaviour problem may be exacerbated if this is suddenly prevented.

The main behaviour problem with Mimi described by her owners occurred at night as they prepared for bed. If Mimi was able to rush in when the bedroom door was first opened, or to take advantage of a lack of supervision while one or other owner went off to clean their teeth, she would leap up onto their bed and void a huge puddle of urine on the covers. This did not happen anywhere else in the house; Mimi was perfectly well house-trained and would ask to be let out to relieve herself when she needed to.

On the face of it, this seems like a fairly easy case to describe. There are, of course, certain suggestions for treatment that anyone with even a little experience in canine behaviour might make, such as not to punish Mimi for urinating, to train her to sit and wait before being allowed in the bedroom, and to make sure she was walked last thing at night before going to bed to try and empty her bladder. However, while punishment by owners is never helpful, other such ostensibly sensible approaches are also often of little value because they are almost impossible to implement, or because they make matters worse initially (extinction burst) and owners become quickly discouraged. For example, introducing a training system whereby Mimi would be expected to learn to wait and sit until the door was opened, and to wait for permission to enter the room and jump up on the bed, would only ensure that she is further frustrated by having to wait and thus would experience an even greater sense of relief when finally allowed into the room and onto the bed. The problem is likely to remain, or probably get worse, with such 're-training'. This case unravels more logically and treatment can be focused much better if it is examined using the EMRA™ approach.

Observations

Mimi became enormously excited at my arrival, as she apparently did with any unusual event in her life. She barked loudly and rushed around between the chair legs under the kitchen table. However, when everyone was calm, she too calmed down and became a very affectionate little dog, who liked nothing more than to be picked up in her lady owner's arms. And if Mrs Kido wasn't available, Mimi was very happy for anyone else to cuddle her. Family mealtimes meant a round of trying to get everyone's attention, pawing at everyone's legs in turn and hoping that someone would pick her up and let her snuggle up behind them on the chair – a warm, dark place of contact where many dogs designed for underground work feel most comfortable.

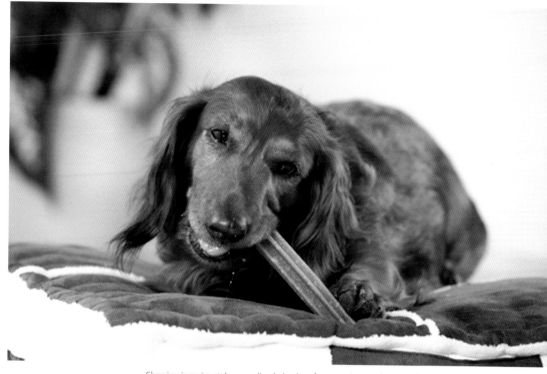

Chewing is an innately rewarding behaviour for most dogs and so providing plenty of chew toys will nearly always improve their Hedonic Budget.

I had already witnessed her reactions to me and to other unfamiliar visitors, both in the short term, and in how long she took to calm down after they had left. Over the course of a couple of days, she had grown used to me in stages. Initially, Mimi had demonstrated a pronounced and prolonged level of excitability, followed by efforts to reassure herself that I was firstly not a threat and then a potential source of attention. On the third day she showed consistently less intense reactions when we met first thing in the morning or after a period of being apart, but still reacted markedly and noisily if I stood up suddenly or moved across the kitchen, for example. If I approached her or tried to lure her to me with a treat, she retreated rapidly and barked loudly at me, pausing only to look either for Mrs Kido, or towards where she usually sat. Finally, by the evening of the third day, I observed a generally calmer acceptance that I was a safe person in Mimi's home and could be trusted if I approached her.

Mimi's reactions to familiar people were perhaps more important. If either of the two nurses from the practice came into the house, as they did quite often to find Dr Kido, Mimi would be delighted and rush up to see them. If they weren't in a hurry, they would fuss her and pet her and she would be happy, and settle quickly if they then put her down or went back out to the surgery. Mimi was used to this and could cope. What she couldn't cope with were the times when they were in a rush and came and went without paying her attention. Then she would bark loudly in her frustration and take quite some time to settle down after they had gone.

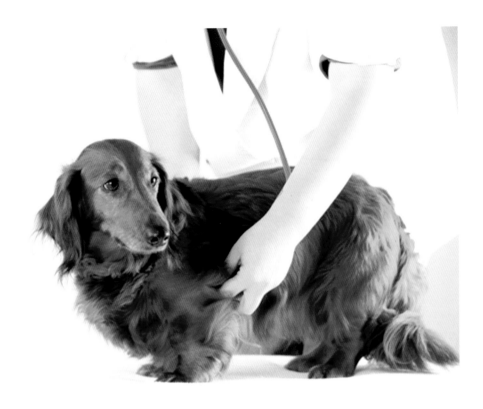

Before being seen by a behaviourist, every dog should be examined by a veterinarian who can assess the presence of any underlying medical cause or influences on the problem behaviour.

More crucial still was the impact that Dr Kido had on his dog's mood state. Like many vets, Dr Kido was very busy with his practice. His activity levels in the kitchen outside the actual surgery hours oscillated between being relaxed and talking to his wife and staff, making phone calls, enjoying tea and sudden bouts of rushing and intense activity if something serious happened in the practice. Sometimes it would only take a phone call with news of an emergency case coming in; at other times it would be one of the nurses rushing in (arousing but ignoring Mimi in the process) and requesting Dr Kido's presence in the surgery to deal with a new client or tend to an animal. For Dr Kido and everyone else, this was a normal part of being a vet in practice whose surgery adjoined his house. Everyone knew to get out of his way in an emergency or at busy times of day. They were used to him suddenly shifting his concentration, and his own emotional state switching instantly from relaxed to near manic on occasion, and had no problems in dealing with it all. Mimi, however, was invariably positioned in her bed right between the surgery entrance and the kitchen, where most of us sat during the day when we were at home, and never knew what was coming next. She simply saw her male owner as a completely unpredictable challenge. One minute he was either neutral or calm and loving, the next, he was the cause of total disruption of her relaxed access to being paid attention, or being part of the family 'heap'. Dr Kido was not a dominating character, and he loved his dog – but when he was busy, his behaviour made her uncertain. Even if he wasn't even looking at her, she immediately tried to resolve the ensuing conflict by adopting an appeasing, comfort-seeking body posture. As a result of this random assault on her routines, Mimi's emotional state oscillated notably around Dr Kido's behaviour, but she was also more sensitised and reactive when Mrs Kido was away and she had to cope with his behaviour without her ultimate safety refuge. As a result, days when Dr Kido was home and busy in and out of the practice almost invariably led to 'pee on the bed nights' for Mimi. She urinated on the bed upstairs in sheer relief at finally getting out of the 'combat zone' of the kitchen/practice interface and becoming safe from the unpredictable random oscillation of Dr Kido's behaviour and, to some extent, that of the nurses.

Emotional Assessment

Just before, during, and just after Mimi's urination on the bed, her emotional state fluctuated considerably and rapidly from one state to another. As shown in Figure 8, just before she entered the bedroom at night, her emotional state was one of miserable frustration. As soon as Mimi entered the bedroom, she tried to leap straight onto the bed,

Figure 8: Assessment of Mimi's emotional state.

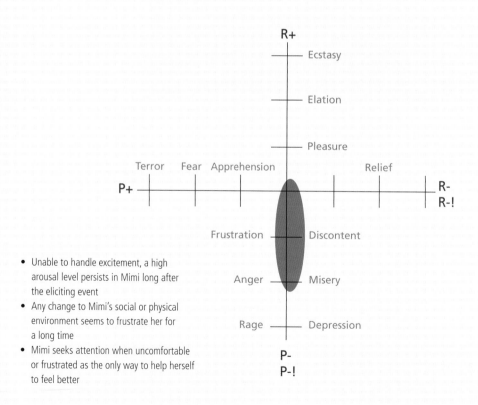

- Unable to handle excitement, a high arousal level persists in Mimi long after the eliciting event
- Any change to Mimi's social or physical environment seems to frustrate her for a long time
- Mimi seeks attention when uncomfortable or frustrated as the only way to help herself to feel better

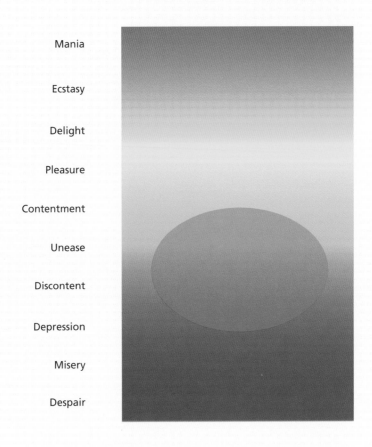

Mania

Ecstasy

Delight

Pleasure

Contentment

Unease

Discontent

Depression

Misery

Despair

Figure 9: Assessment of Mimi's mood state.

which, in Japanese style, was low to the ground. When she got to this ultimate place of relaxation and safety, she experienced an overwhelming feeling of relief, driving her emotional state into a mix of relief and pleasure, an emotional state very different from her day-to-day mood state. The bladder emptying, I suggest, was involuntary, a reaction similar to that which a dog or a person might have when suddenly terrified by something but in very much the opposite sense emotionally. In addition, voiding of the bladder is itself internally rewarding and served to enhance the pleasure of the moment even further.

Mood State Assessment

Mimi's general mood was in a state of oscillating extremes throughout the day but was generally unhappy and miserable, as shown in Figure 9. For much of the time, when she was either alone or with Mrs Kido, she was quite calm and, when she went out for her short walks, she became more relaxed and was happy to meet other people and dogs. But the minute anyone entered her daytime 'inner sanctum' of the living room and kitchen, she immediately became highly excited and her reactive barking and excitable rushing around continued long afterwards. Her mood remained elevated long after the person had gone away. If they stayed and she didn't know them, she would become obsessed about getting their attention and tried perpetually, it seemed, to reassure herself that they were available on demand to fuss her, and maybe pick her up and cuddle her. This was a sustained effort in an attempt to maintain her mood in a more positive state and was one of the few opportunities available to her. However, whether the visitors stayed or went, Mimi's level of arousal was marked and persisted for a long time, as opposed to the normal shorter-term emotional response followed by a calming down that one might expect in most dogs. By the time she went to bed at night on such days, she would be highly agitated and desperate to get to her one place of ultimate relaxation and safety in the bedroom upstairs, and to be alone again with Mrs Kido.

On quieter days, and notably those with no visitors, Mimi's mood wouldn't become so agitated and she would jump on the bed at night in calmer mood and be far less likely to empty her bladder. However, these days were becoming ever less frequent. Her mood state was generally miserable and depressed (Figure 9), and the opportunities presented for finding relief by going to bed at night were fast becoming her habitual way of relaxing and elevating her mood.

Reinforcement Assessment

In the previous cases we discussed the behavioural characteristics of different types of dog, as the presence or absence of opportunities to carry out type-favoured behaviours especially will have a great influence on the dog's general mood state. Such opportunities can be usefully represented in the form of a 'Hedonic Budget'. Various innately

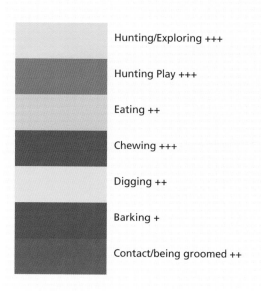

Figure 10: Hedonic Budget of a typical 3-year-old Miniature Long-haired Dachshund.

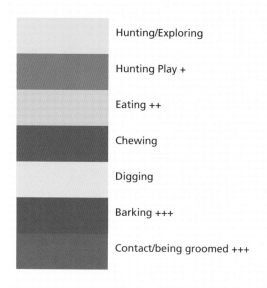

Figure 11: Mimi's Hedonic Budget.

39

rewarding behaviours, such as chewing, drinking, social interaction, elimination, sleep, etc., are clearly important to all dogs. They are vital for the maintenance of a normal state of resting contentment and can also be usefully incorporated into a basic Hedonic Budget representation. The presence or absence, or the level, of such opportunities in any dog's lifestyle is of crucial relevance to the establishment of their general mood state and behaviour. Analysing the Hedonic Budget often very usefully helps us to see why and how a dog responds emotionally and behaviourally in any given situation when it becomes aroused, and what it may attempt to do to maintain a comfortable feeling of wellbeing. It is therefore also crucial to consider at this stage which of the rewarding opportunities/activities that are important to the dog in question are in short supply, or missing altogether from their Hedonic Budget, and so might be utilised in a behaviour modification programme.

Breed-specific behaviours important for a Miniature Long-haired Dachshund in addition to, or at greater levels than, those applying to all dogs, include hunting, digging, shaking prey or toys in substitute play, going to 'ground' when resting or sleeping and social contact with their owners (after Coppinger and Coppinger, 2001). A typical ideal Hedonic Budget showing a few of these behavioural opportunities for a Miniature Long-haired Dachshund is shown in Figure 10, and Mimi's in Figure 11. It is clear that Mimi's Hedonic Budget was far from ideal on most days and this clearly helps to explain her depressed countenance, her emotional reactivity in response to unusual events around her and the prolonged effect that such changes had on her mood state.

In terms of reinforcement assessment, therefore, it is clear that if there were no emotional benefit to Mimi for voiding her bladder on the bed, even involuntarily, then the behaviour would never have been established or repeated, nor withstood any efforts to remove it. Any treatment must first uncouple the feelings of success or relief that have become learned and established at carrying out the behaviour. In many cases, only then can one establish opportunities for the dog to carry out alternative, but equally successful or relief-bringing, behaviours, which then themselves can be reinforced and established in those circumstances or in any particular environment.

Previous Attempts at Treatment

While many owners would simply have disbarred the dog from the bedroom, keeping her out was not an option for Mrs Kido, who, like many owners of small (and sometimes big!) dogs, liked the warmth and security of a dog on the bed at night. In any case, having already tried both leaving Mimi in her usual daytime rest bed downstairs at night and restraining her to it in the bedroom with a leash tied to a chair, the owners had found that she barked and howled continuously and so they had given up in order to get some sleep!

Mimi's problem was persisting and steadily worsening, despite the owners' attempts to resolve it at the time, i.e. to deal with her emotionality and behaviour at the time of the likely urination. They had tried telling her off, tried to distract and reward her for going on to the bed without wetting it, and tried delaying her access to the bed. None of these tactics had altered her desperate mood at bedtime and so none of these attempts had produced any positive effect. The reinforcement for the urination was the internal sense of relief that Mimi felt after a bad mood state day, and did not result from any consequential or subsequent external factors. Obviously, punishing her or telling her off in the bedroom would only be likely to make her afraid at the same time as relieved, causing a real mix-up of emotions and lead-

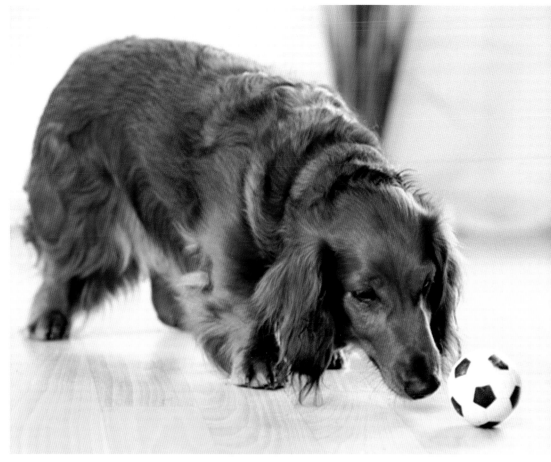

A dog that cannot fulfil their ideal Hedonic Budget with normally rewarding activities may become depressed, inactive and lethargic, engage in the opportunities that are available to higher levels than normal (e.g. eat more), or engage in behaviour in ways that make them feel better but which are potentially problematic (e.g. circling).

ing to a worsening of the problem. Trying to calm her or reward her at the time she was on the bed may also only have enhanced her sense of reward and relief and so further reinforce the aroused emotional state. In fact, the internal reinforcement of Mimi getting to the bed was so strong that there was probably nothing at all that the owners could do at the time to calm her or improve her behaviour.

It was clear that Mimi was very used to going to bed with her owners, and that to advise them to do what to some might be the obvious suggestion, i.e. make her sleep in a bed or pen down-

stairs, was therefore going to be unacceptable. It was not acceptable to Mrs Kido, and would also be unpleasant for Mimi, who would be further distressed and aroused by such a change, may start urinating wherever she was put instead, and probably develop other problems, such as inappropriate defecation, or howling and whining. Such tactics may be successful in other circumstances with different dogs in different mood states and with different owners, but this is the point about not applying standardised approaches to treatment even if they are sensible or successful for some. If the owners don't like the ideas, and won't apply them anyway, the behaviour therapist must devise approaches that accommodate their wishes. If the therapist advises that the dog should just 'put up with changes and get used to it', and that the owners must simply deal with the unpleasant consequences of their dog's distress, then treatment is often doomed to failure, because the owners will quickly give up and ignore the advice. It's no good then blaming them for not following advice that they are unable to apply. The EMRA™ approach allows cases to be approached far more sensitively, and takes account of the specific emotionality of the dog and needs of the owners.

Treatment

It was established quickly that there was little the owners could do at the time they actually went to bed if Mimi was already in a sufficiently distressed mood. Therefore treatment was initially to be aimed almost entirely at maintaining her mood state at a less aroused, more even level during the day, so that she would be calmer and able to manage her own emotions at bedtime. This involved further scrutiny of how her days would pass, both in terms of her social relationships with all the people in her life, including visitors, and her opportunities for stimulation such as play, chewing toys, walks and her routines.

Clearly we couldn't expect Dr Kido to restructure his practice hours, nor move out of his surgery, but we could manage Mimi's exposure to the consequences of living in the middle of it all. Mimi's bed was to be moved away from the passageway between the entrance leading to the practice and the kitchen, and positioned on the other side of the kitchen, closer to the back door and on the side where Mrs Kido sat relaxing or preparing family meals. Then Mimi would have access to her in the event of unusual disturbances and would be out of the direct firing line of commotion within the practice. She could still bark at whatever was happening but would calm down more quickly from her protected bed and with Mrs Kido close by to reassure her. Mimi would still have access to Dr Kido when he was calm, and to the nurses arriving if they had time, but if things got suddenly busy, Mimi could swiftly retreat to safety instead of being caught in the crossfire with her route to her day bed and Mrs Kido blocked.

Improving the Hedonic Budget

To achieve this, I asked Mrs Kido to establish a routine of regular exercise and play outdoors for Mimi in frequent short sessions in the yard. I had noticed that while Mimi had her comfort rag doll toy in her bed and occasionally held it in her mouth, or nestled close up to it, she had no other chew toys. This was because the Kidos were concerned about her 'rather delicate teeth and gums' and consequently fed soft foods to avoid provoking injury or damage. With Dr Kido's agreement I gave her a tooth-cleaning, more easily crumbled, bone-shaped chew toy. She immediately took this to her bed and sat and chewed intently until it was all gone! Interestingly, she was not only calm when the nurses or Dr Kido came and went around her, whatever their mood state, while she was chewing, but she also remained in a very relaxed mood long after she had finished.

It sounds obvious, but dogs need to run about, socialise, play and chew every day. As we have discussed already, these activities are rewarding just to do, with no need for an outcome or independent reinforcement. As a result, just doing them maintains a dog's mood state at normal,

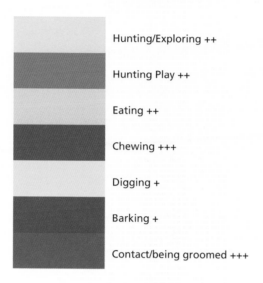

Hunting/Exploring ++

Hunting Play ++

Eating ++

Chewing +++

Digging +

Barking +

Contact/being groomed +++

Figure 12: Mimi's Hedonic Budget after starting therapy.

balances out their brain reward chemistry, and makes them 'happier' and less sensitive to other events when aroused emotionally. If dogs don't get sufficient opportunity to carry out such behaviours, then their mood state can either become depressed if they are introverted characters, or easily aroused by other events and remaining so for longer if they are extroverts like Mimi.

All of these suggestions were designed to diversify and improve Mimi's Hedonic Budget (see Figure 12) and so to elevate her mood state to a normal level of resting contentment for her type/breed and age. This was coupled with a common-sense suggestion of not playing with her or exciting her deliberately in the half-hour or so before everyone went to bed. In this way we hoped to prevent the build-up of the mood state that Mimi had often experienced at bed time which then led directly to the big wet patches and late night bed cover changes! Of course Mimi was

safe to be allowed back on the bed after one episode of urination as she was then emotionally relieved and her bladder was empty, and so she had always been allowed back after the covers were changed!

Results

The approach to treatment of the behaviour problem by managing Mimi's mood state worked perfectly, and surprisingly rapidly, and was accompanied by excellent observable general improvements in Mimi's level of arousal and emotional response to the arrival of visitors and other unexpected events (see Figure 13). Over the course of my 5-day stay, Mimi learned how to manage her own general behaviour in the kitchen in a much more restrained manner and clearly benefited from the increased opportunity to per-

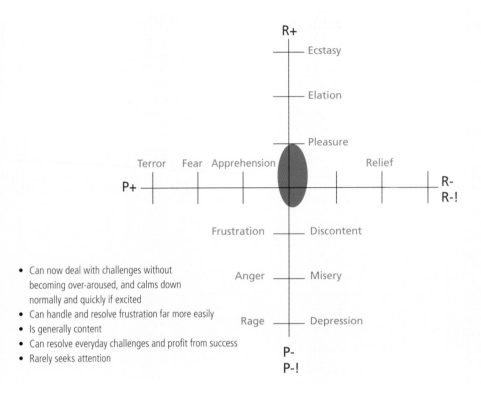

- Can now deal with challenges without becoming over-aroused, and calms down normally and quickly if excited
- Can handle and resolve frustration far more easily
- Is generally content
- Can resolve everyday challenges and profit from success
- Rarely seeks attention

Figure 13: Assessment of Mimi's emotional state after behaviour therapy.

Figure 14: Assessment of Mimi's mood state after therapy.

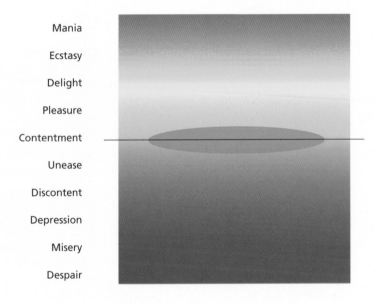

form many more 'Dachshund type' activities during the day in the beneficial routine organised by Mrs Kido. Mimi enjoyed contact with the nurses at calm times and Dr Kido when he was least likely to rush off suddenly, and learned to relax in her new day bed, which also served as her den. She sat contentedly in there near Mrs Kido, as opposed to trying constantly to get on her lap, often chewing a chew with such concentration that she failed to notice if a visitor arrived or Dr Kido rushed into the kitchen. She was, quite simply, a much happier dog (see Figure 14).

On the second night after the treatment to adjust her mood state began, there was no urination when she went to bed and she was noticebly very relaxed, and slept well and comfortably, according to the owners. There had been no 'extinction burst' in the response to treatment when I left the Kido household, and by the time I left for the UK about 10 days later, the owners reported that Mimi was consistently going to bed in a much calmer state and hadn't urinated once.

This case presents an excellent example of just how vital it is to assess an animal's lifestyle and resulting mood state when approaching any behaviour problem. In this example, raising the level of resting contentment to be more in keeping with what Mimi needed as an individual precluded any need to target her emotional state or the resulting behaviour at the time she presented with the urination problem (see Figure 10). As a result, Mimi and her owners could enjoy much happier lives in return for relatively little effort and few changes to their busy routines, as opposed to protracted efforts at behaviour therapy that might try and target the dog's emotional state and behaviour at the time of the problem. By addressing Mimi's lifestyle and resultant mood state, everyone could now go to bed at night and relax, safe in the knowledge that the bed would stay dry after they entered the bedroom!

CASE HISTORY 4: 'Rage syndrome'

DOG:
Bracken, red Cocker Spaniel
AGE:
15 months
SEX:
Male
PROBLEM:
Snapping/growling when frustrated

In this case example we refer to a behavioural case history and discuss how a so-called 'diagnosis' of 'rage syndrome' can be reassessed more accurately using the EMRA™ model and how treatment can be devised far more effectively.

Bracken is an energetic, lively, playful and enthusiastic bouncy young Cocker Spaniel, owned since he was 9 weeks of age by a young middle-aged couple. They researched his breed very carefully before searching out the best breeder they could find: one who raised her pups in the home, who clearly understood and loved her dogs and her breed, and where they could see Bracken's mother. They raised the question of 'rage syndrome' with her and were reassured that while there was some concern about red, and perhaps other solid-coloured Cockers, none of her breeding line, nor the stud she had engaged with her bitch to produce Bracken and his litter, had ever shown any propensity for aggression.

Bracken was chirpy right from the start and soon settled in, went to puppy classes as the breeder had advised, and grew into a very pleasant and well-behaved young dog. At 1 year old, he was into anything and everything and had never been aggressive with other dogs or the owners' young nephews when they come to stay, though he

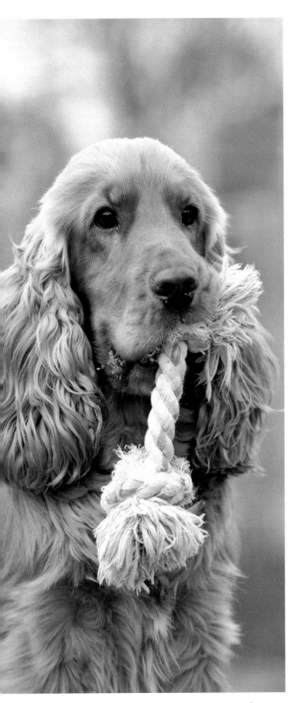

Even though we now know it does not exist, some owners fear a so-called 'diagnosis' of incurable 'Cocker rage syndrome' if their spaniel shows the slightest signs of aggression, such as growling to defend toys or food.

always drew the line when he had had enough disturbance from them, or at rough play from other larger dogs. He was reported as being quite quick to protest at such times and quite emphatic, and to give out a sudden 'snap growl' to signal 'game over'. The message seemed clear enough to other dogs, and they usually walked away quickly. One of the owners' nephews also realised that 'no means no' after one short lesson when Bracken told him a second time after he carried on demanding to play, and he felt the dog's hot breath on his hand as he 'snapped' at him more emphatically. The owners witnessed the whole event and described Bracken's behaviour as completely r easonable in the circumstances, and viewed his snap as a very quick but very controlled response to unreasonable interference. Teeth didn't touch skin and the nephew simply got up off the floor and ran off, leaving Bracken to go and rest in his basket. A few minutes later he was outside playing with the children again quite happily.

So why were the owners concerned? They felt that Bracken's tendency to behave in this way in response to contact that he either didn't want from the start, or that went on too long for him, or that he found too rough, was perhaps increasing of late. They called the breeder and she advised them to keep an eye on Bracken and to try not to provoke him into reacting. She also advised them to seek help immediately if they were ever concerned that his temper was on too much of a knife-edge for their safety, or if they became worried that he might bite someone or get into a dog fight. However, the owners decided that they would rather not wait for any disasters and sought our help in case he had the awful-sounding 'rage syndrome' developing now that he was an adolescent.

We always shudder when we hear the words 'Cocker Spaniel' and anything to do with aggression in the same sentence because we know that the words 'rage syndrome' are following not far behind and will be on the lips of the owner, the breeder, the referring vet and anyone else concerned. The first job in cases such as Bracken's is to dispel the dreadful myth that the dog is suffering with some incurable genetic affliction that is likely to cause injury and pain to his owners on a random and serious basis for all time, and then try to deal properly with the problem at hand. We believe that the whole condition was a fabrication from the start or, at best, a smokescreen set up by early behaviourists who didn't know what to do with aggressive Cockers or how to explain what was going on. The result has been that owners and countless responsible breeders of this fabulous breed of dog all walk in fear of the 'curse of rage syndrome' and become enormously concerned if their dog so much as growls, and panic if they happen to lose their temper one day.

Meeting Bracken and his Owners

When I visited the owners, I found that Bracken, just like so many other so-called 'raging' Cockers I have met over the years, was a fabulous little dog. He was full of enthusiasm and the tough spirit that befits an energetic working gundog. He had the innate desirable ability to respond quickly to changing events; for example, when his toy disappeared into a thicket and his way was barred he simply redoubled his efforts to get to it either by bashing his way through the thorns of a gorse bush or by running around and trying to get it from a different angle.

Having made friends by feeding him a couple of treats and throwing his ball for him when we all first met, I decided to investigate whether his temper would snap into a rage when he was thwarted from his working intentions when he was at his most excited and motivated. This is only recommended for those like me who desire to see where the limits lie in this so-called raging breed. Please 'do not do this at home' or,

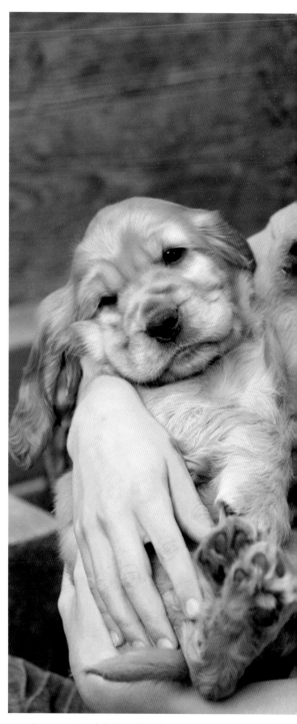

Even experienced, dedicated breeders are unable to guarantee the future behaviour of their puppies unconditionally.

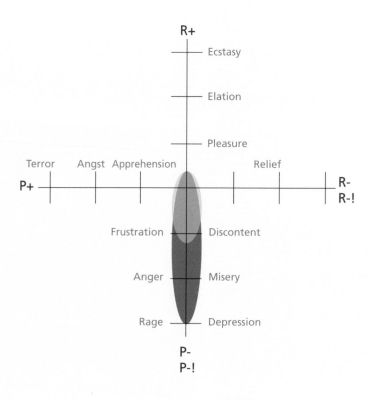

Figure 15: Assessment of Bracken's emotional state: frustration.
Figure 16: The emotional state of a raging dog.

indeed, with any dog. So I simply grabbed Bracken and picked him up as he rushed past me on his way to get his ball out of a gorse thicket. He wriggled hard but he kept his eye intently on where he had been heading and, when I still wouldn't let go, yes … he did what any dog may do when he is 'attacked' at such a moment. He growled! But it wasn't at me, it was simply an expression of his frustration at not being able to do what he wanted to do. At no point did I think he would go on to growl at me or bite me. And when I still wouldn't let go, he just wriggled more and growled a higher pitched oscillating frustrated growl, and then he just gave up, went still and looked at me. Game over, no problem, no rage. I put him down, and he went and retrieved his ball, and brought it to me to throw again.

Emotional Assessment

Our assessment of Bracken using the EMRA™ model is that Bracken lets you know how he feels at all times. He will growl to tell the world what he is feeling when he is excited and frustrated, but he is very capable of restraining his emotions and responses even at such a time. If the owners don't like being growled at, then obviously they shouldn't frustrate him at such times, but the point is that on the emotional scale, Bracken is only frustrated (see Figure 15) by being denied. He isn't angry and doesn't fly into a rage, at least not in this test. If he were less restrained, his emotional assessment would have been depicted as

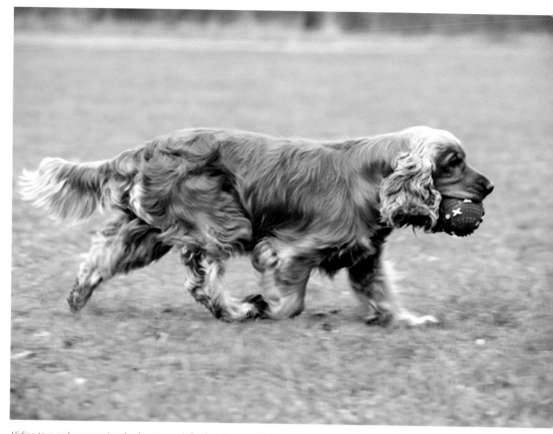

Hiding toys and encouraging the dog to search for them is an excellent way of integrating problem-solving tasks into the everyday life of dogs from breeds that have the traditional role of flushing out game, and is especially important in a non-working domestic setting.

in Figure 16. Hence Bracken's owners were immediately reassured that Bracken's capacity for emotional restraint and focus on the job in hand were excellent, and these were actually two important qualities for a good working Cocker.

Evolution and Brain Chemistry of Hunting Dogs

To try to discover what is going on when dogs 'lose their temper', or how well they can restrain their emotions and reactions when aroused, we should look first at 'dog the hunter' and the evolution of working types of dog. Mammalian predators hunt in what is called a motor pattern, a genetically based sequence of behaviour. Once they have searched their environment and caught sight of their quarry, a pattern is invoked: eye–stalk–chase–pounce/grab/bite–dissect/kill. Hunting is a 'self-rewarding' activity in that performing the behaviour itself releases a high level of neurotransmitters such as dopamine that are associated with feelings of reward (and thus reinforcement) in the brains of predators, although outwardly they show little emotion while they approach, attack and kill their prey. Most of the time, of course, their prey escapes, but even without fulfilling the final step of biting and killing the prey, the hunter obtains a huge reward simply by

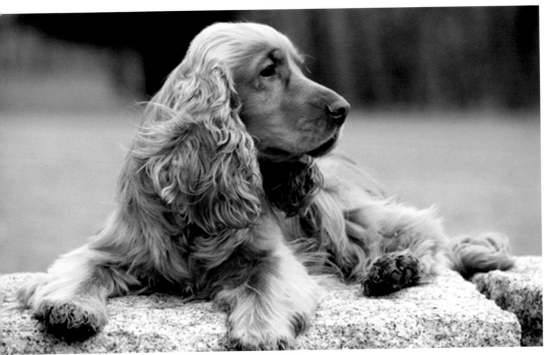

Living with an owner who fails to understand the emotional and behavioural needs of a working gundog type can be very frustrating for some Cocker Spaniels in a non-working setting, and may eventually lead to the dog becoming angry if frustrated over some minor issue. But there is no scientific evidence to suggest that this is a psychological or physiological disorder that can be inherited, and many dogs respond very well indeed to being given more challenges and working gundog-style activities to pursue.

commencing the 'eye' fix of the prey, and then going through any section of their innate predatory sequence. The behaviour is rewarded and thus reinforced at every stage and at every attempt and thus is highly resistant to failure.

Dogs have evolved from the ancestral predator, the wolf (via the village dog), with some or all of this hunting behaviour sequence retained in most, but deliberately modified by humans into specific useful forms in certain types by reducing, deleting or enhancing aspects of this motor pattern (see Coppinger and Coppinger, 2001). Indeed, the fact

that aspects of this predatory sequence can be selected for underlines the fact that it is genetically based. For example, one of the earliest uses for dogs that humans bred in them was the ability to herd sheep. To do this, they use the 'eye–stalk–chase' components, but the bite/kill has been selected out so that, when herding, dogs do not actually attack the sheep, but simply move them. Of course some young collies do 'nip' the heels of the sheep, which is an inhibited bite and a 'fault' that can usually be trained out of the dog. Any dogs that actually attack and bite the sheep are

* The progress of the domestication of dogs from wolves can be viewed on DVD (3x 3 hours) of Ray Coppinger's extraordinary seminar 'Of Wolves and Dogs', held in the UK, available online at www.pneville.com. The DVDs of Professor Coppinger's other UK seminars: 'The Emotions, Intelligence and Behaviour of Dogs' and 'Mexico City Dump Dogs' are also available at the same website.

usually not kept for work and not bred from, hence their more serious working 'fault' is removed from the gene pool, and this is exactly how selective breeding for proficiency at any task is established in the population. Dogs bred to guard sheep, such as the Maremma, do not show the initial 'eye' behaviour in the company of sheep, and so these dogs are able to be left alone with flocks to protect them against attacks by wolves, their very own ancestors.

Some types have had the enthusiastic stalk–chase parts of the hunting sequence enhanced and these have been shaped through selective breeding for performance to be the flushers of game when humans go hunting. Spaniels are a prime example of this type of enthusiastic modified predator, and they also often make good retrievers of the game we kill. Retrievers have similarly had the 'grab' part of the predatory sequence enhanced by selective breeding. They reliably eye–stalk–chase–GRAB, but then bring the prey to their handler or owner because the bite/dissect end parts of the original sequence have been markedly reduced or removed from the gene pool and they don't really know what else to do! Such dogs have also proved highly useful to humans as hunting dogs.

The crucial point in all of this is that whatever aspects of this original hunting motor pattern have been selected for over thousands of generations by humans, every dog gets a huge reward out of just being able to perform whatever parts of that sequence they were bred to do as a working dog. The converse of that pleasure is that they can experience intense frustration when they can't perform those behaviours enough (see Blum et al., 1996). In recent times, of course, dogs of all types are far more likely to have been selected for breeding because of their looks in a show ring rather than their working ability. While most adapt quite happily to a more sedentary lifestyle as pets, with an occasional opportunity to express their parts of that critical hunting sequence through chasing balls and sending squirrels up trees, or fixing the cat with that collie 'eye', some types and some breeds, and some individuals in those types and breeds, adapt better than others. The Cocker Spaniel, the archetypal pretty small- to medium-sized playful house pet for a modern life-style, is simply a breed in which more individuals don't seem to adapt to this less active and less stimulating lifestyle so well. It's all very logical, and ought to lead us to think rather more carefully about so-called 'rage syndrome' and aggression generally in Cocker Spaniels, and to consider their lifestyle and behaviour more from their emotional point of view.

The History of So-called Rage Syndrome

The 'Rage Syndrome' label was first described in the USA in the 1970s and then introduced to the UK by a well-known behaviourist in the early 1980s. However, it has never been proven to exist as a heritable syndrome in Cockers or any other breed, either in the USA or in the UK. Despite several scientific investigations into possible links with epilepsy at Liverpool Veterinary School, investigations at Cambridge Veterinary School by veterinary ethologists, several surveys by breed clubs and private investigations by concerned individuals involved with the breed, no abnormalities have ever been identified in any behavioural, genetic or post-mortem studies. Yet the whole concept of rage syndrome has become repeated so often by so many that it is now believed to be an accepted 'condition' in much of the behaviour/veterinary world. The only end result is that some colours, and especially the reds, of a really super breed of dog have been maligned and tarred with a reputation that isn't justified according to any

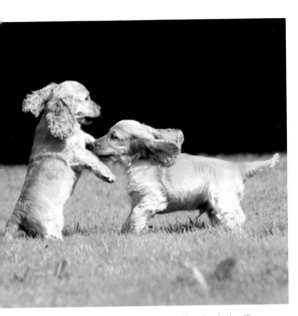

Despite several investigations, there is still no hard scientific evidence to support the description of an inherited condition of 'Cocker rage', and yet some breeders, veterinarians, trainers and behaviourists will make a 'diagnosis' of incurable 'rage syndrome' if they see an angry or aggressive Cocker.

scientific evidence. The vast majority of behaviour problems, even dramatic ones, are not clinical diseases, and the tendency to view them and treat them as such should be resisted.

Modern-day pet Cockers have the simple misfortune to descend from a highly intelligent working breed with a high demand for work and stimulation that simply isn't available in most pet owners' homes. There is often simply not enough opportunity for the dog to solve problems in such homes, and in particular the types of problem that go with quick thinking and doing the job that Cockers were bred to do – which is to hunt game, flush it out and then retrieve it after it has been shot. Loved to death and given all the best food, treats and fuss, and veterinary care in the world, they simply don't get to do what they are designed to, and the types of games they may get to play are neither good enough nor frequent

enough models of their working needs to satisfy them. As a result, some Cockers can suffer from immense frustration in home environments, but they do restrain themselves admirably until some minor event proves to be the straw that breaks the camel's back and then they fly off the handle. Being tough gundogs underneath those floppy ears, they attack well and so, like any provoked dog in a highly aroused state, they can be dangerous when their temper does finally break (see Figure 16).

Just imagine if you were a highly trained mathematician but weren't given a computer or even a pen and paper to exercise your skills. Or maybe a highly trained, fit long-distance runner who was only ever allowed to run for short distances in the garden. The impact on your general mood, even though you may be living in a 5-star hotel with all the comfort and fine food you could want, would be enormous. Of course on most days you might just be able to behave in a civilised fashion. Introverts may just give up and become depressed, but supposing you were the human equivalent of a Cocker Spaniel – an extrovert by birth? Your mood may also be restrained most of the time as you got excited about even small infrequent opportunities to do something new, and these just about kept you happy most of the time. But on bad days, if you were rubbed up the wrong way, it is highly likely that you would instantly lose your temper with whoever happened to be nearby! Does that mean that you too could be diagnosed as being emotionally dysfunctional, as having rage syndrome? Or would you prefer someone to look at the bigger picture of your whole lifestyle and its impact on your mood, rather than just your occasional outbursts?

So it is with Cockers, we believe. Far from being reactive, incipiently moody, dysfunctional psychopaths, we feel that these dogs are often immensely self-restrained in such emotionally limiting circumstances. Cockers have the misfortune to look cute and so may be pampered, and are often kept as pets for older people who may not stimulate them or exercise them much. But such owners may spend a lot of time with them and so they are perhaps even more susceptible to the consequences of any serious sudden loss of temper. This is, of course, often made all the more serious because of the age of such owners. It is perhaps something of a miracle that more Cockers, and indeed other high-energy working breeds forced to lead a dull pet lifestyle, don't explode with anger or rage sometimes. Referring to some earlier works on this subject, some authors describe that rage syndrome has indeed occasionally been reported in other breeds. It's surely no surprise to find that these individuals, for the most part, are also from traditional working breeds who have been denied the chance to do their 'work' in their domestic home, such as the Golden Retriever, Pyrenean and Bernese Mountain Dog, and, in the USA, the odd yard-bound German Shepherd Dog or two.

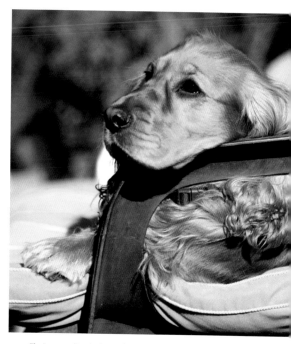

Their appealing looks and convenient size in a domestic setting mean that some Cocker Spaniels unfortunately end up with more sedentary or senior owners and are forced to live a life that is neither sufficiently stimulating nor emotionally fulfilling for them.

No Pathology

The real point that totally undermines a 'diagnosis' of rage syndrome as a pathological disorder is surely that attacks cited in Cockers are always aimed at someone, and don't just happen spontaneously. No one ever came home to find their dog midway through savaging the curtains, the table or even the cat. It is people who are the source of the final straw in the frustration of the dog. But instead of leading behaviourists to question the inherited pathological explanation for 'rage', this simple syndrome-discrediting observation led them to view quick-tempered Cockers as having some kind of very sharp dominance aggression, (another now long discredited diag-

nostic description). And so they treated these cases with so-called 'dominance reduction' programmes based on 'Learn to Earn' or 'Nothing in Life is Free' tactics. These approaches made the things that the dog liked suddenly totally unavailable, or at least much less available, and so they naturally became even more frustrated and reacted more intensely more often. With an escalation in attacks, the behaviourist and vets alike thus pointed to a growing pathology and recommended euthanasia without further delay. Sadly this simply further perpetuated the myth that such Cockers were dangerously dysfunctional as a result of some heritable condition, and that the rage was due to some as yet unidentified clinical influence.

As a result of all of this, over the years far too many stroppy, or even normally reactive extrovert,

Cockers have been diagnosed as having rage syndrome and many even euthanased as incurable, as 'better do it now before it gets worse' cases. This has been and continues to be one of the biggest shames of the behaviour profession, because these dogs are apparently not clinically abnormal at all. With a little attention to their circumstances or, in the case of elderly people, a little better advice about the lack of emotional suitability of Cockers for a more sedentary lifestyle, these dogs would not behave so dangerously and dramatically.

Mood Assessment

If we are not to see this type of explosive behaviour as some incurable syndrome, how are we to see it, and how are we to approach or, better, prevent the problems associated with loss of temper in the domestic setting? As far back as the mid-1990s, COAPE behaviourists began to treat these cases in a way that we now know as one based on mood state adjustment and achieved some great results. This approach involves first assessing the dog's estimated Hedonic Budget for their type/breed/age/sex, etc. (see Figure 17a) and comparing this with the one they currently experience (see Figure 17b). This helped us to expose any major deficiencies and thus formed the basis of our advice to the owners about how to improve Bracken's lifestyle and sustain him in the happiest general mood possible. Plotting Bracken's general mood also enables us to demonstrate the level of mood adjustment required through improvements in his lifestyle (see Figure 18).

We thus set about providing resolvable frustrations in Bracken's life, using enrichment, in the form of removing the food bowl and hiding all his food, then putting it in foraging toys such as Activity Balls, Buster Cubes, Busy Buddy toys, etc.

His owners were shown how to lay scent trails for him to follow around the home and garden and it was suggested that they train Bracken to the gun, even if they themselves were not hunters. Once he had been trained, perhaps a shooting friend or someone from the gundog training club nearby would appreciate his services. It was also suggested that they walk Bracken off lead as much as possible in more places in the New Forest where they lived, and generally introduce routines of activity and problem-solving for him at home involving hiding toys and basic response and trick training. Such efforts alleviated the reward deficit of dogs in many of our cases in the late 1990s, and crucially made them appreciate their down time, as the opportunity to rest at home, rather than seething with frustration and then exploding from time to time (see Figure 19). In most cases, no more attacks ever occurred. In others, notable reductions in the frequency and severity of attacks, and a great improvement in the calm-restoring distractibility, of so-called raging dogs was achieved not only with Cockers, but also with other short-fused and apparently unpredictably aggressive dogs.

Reinforcement Assessment

The emotional assessment of such dogs at the time of an attack shows anger, not rage. The mood state is one of smouldering dissatisfaction, and the reinforcement assessment for the attack is the internal relief it brings against a backdrop of the stress of a continually frustrating lifestyle (see Figure 18). Lashing out at one identifiable source of that frustration makes the dog feel better, and that in itself can become addictive, which is why such cases often get worse if left untreated. These Cockers may not show it but they are hugely stressed by their lifestyles, and so the aim

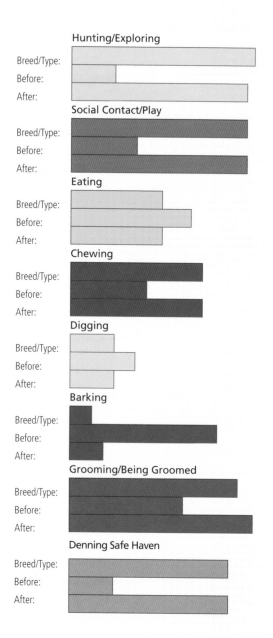

Hunting/Exploring

Breed/Type:
Before:
After:

Social Contact/Play

Breed/Type:
Before:
After:

Eating

Breed/Type:
Before:
After:

Chewing

Breed/Type:
Before:
After:

Digging

Breed/Type:
Before:
After:

Barking

Breed/Type:
Before:
After:

Grooming/Being Groomed

Breed/Type:
Before:
After:

Denning Safe Haven

Breed/Type:
Before:
After:

Figure 17: Hedonic Budgets
(a) Bre-Typ: Cocker Spaniel breed-typical Hedonic Budget
(b) Before: Bracken's initial Hedonic Budget
(c) After: Bracken's Hedonic Budget after treatment

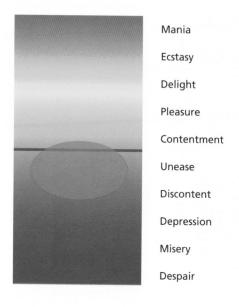

Mania

Ecstasy

Delight

Pleasure

Contentment

Unease

Discontent

Depression

Misery

Despair

Figure 18: Assessment of Bracken's mood state before therapy.

of treatment is to attempt to redress this through lifestyle adjustment rather than confrontation or attempts to treat at the time of the emotional outburst. At such times, owners are advised to remove themselves to a safe place behind a door as quickly as possible from the dog. They should wait for the dog to calm down before attracting them out into the garden and trying to engage them in retrieving games that engage the predatory behaviour appropriately and safely.

Outcome

Applied to Bracken, the EMRA™ approach and Hedonic Budget improvement rapidly produced excellent results (Figure 17c). Bracken has never so much as looked angry at home or in the forest

Case History 5: Separation-related problem

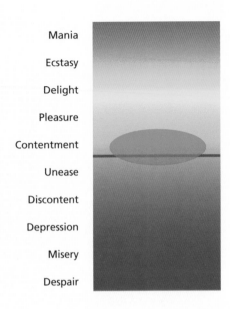

Mania

Ecstasy

Delight

Pleasure

Contentment

Unease

Discontent

Depression

Misery

Despair

Figure 19: Assessment of Bracken's mood state after the commencement of behaviour therapy.

since treatment began. He is either active doing something or enjoying being groomed and fussed, or he is resting quietly (see Figure 19). A little bomb he may be, by virtue of having been bred to do a job that requires reactivity and persistent enthusiasm, and perhaps he might have exploded as an expected emotional consequence if he had been frustrated for great lengths of time. But, by understanding this, we have ensured that he is never so frustrated or close to reacting explosively, and we have defused him permanently and safely and he should now have a long enjoyable life with two caring owners.

DOG:
Cassie, Schnauzer
AGE:
8 months
SEX:
Entire female
PROBLEM:
Separation-related problem

Jane and Stephen sought help for Cassie as she could not be left alone in the house without noisy consequences. They were not very sure of the extent of the problem but were aware that something was wrong as a result of Cassie's highly effusive welcoming behaviour and past experiences (now infrequent) of house soiling when she was left. They felt the problem started very early on in her life with them, although they couldn't be precise. Cassie had been easy to house-train, therefore it came as a surprise when Jane found that she had soiled indoors when left alone, even though she had been adequately exercised. The soiling was mainly limited to the hall and kitchen but occasionally occurred in the bedroom and was not punished by her owners. The behaviour had stopped except on very rare occasions. Jane said that she knew that this could indicate a potential for Cassie to have a separation-related problem.

Cassie's excessive greeting behaviour, even after short absences, was one of the main causes for concern as she would enter a highly aroused state, jumping, whining and 'crying' when reunited with her owners, sometimes for as long as 20 minutes. It was not known whether she was vocalising when left alone as their neighbour in the attached house is very deaf and although they live in a cul-de-sac, the neighbour on the other side is not close and has not heard any noise. Cassie constantly follows her owners everywhere around the house. She may appear to be asleep but immediately gets up if they move. Although she is not attention-seeking in a pushy way, she likes close physical contact with them much of the time.

The problem time for her owners now is when Stephen works nights. He spends the day with Cassie and leaves home to go to work at 5 pm. Jane arrives home between 6.30 and 7.00 pm, and it is this 1.5- to 2-hour period that is causing concern. Stephen's night shifts are irregular, only about three nights per month. Also, if Jane needs to go shopping, Cassie has to be dropped off with her parents because she becomes very distressed if left at home or in the car. She does not appear to become particularly distressed or anxious during her owners' preparations to leave the house and she has never been destructive in their absence.

Cassie has also become rather lacking in confidence when out and about, sometimes unwilling to pass a bus queue, for example, and she backs away when strangers speak to her, which is another cause for concern. She is interested in other dogs and will approach them excitedly but doesn't have any 'dog friends'. Although Jane and Stephen have no children, theirs is a busy household with regular visitors with whom Cassie is comfortable.

Video Investigation

A week prior to my visit I lent a video camera to Jane and Stephen and asked them to leave it running when Stephen left to go to work.

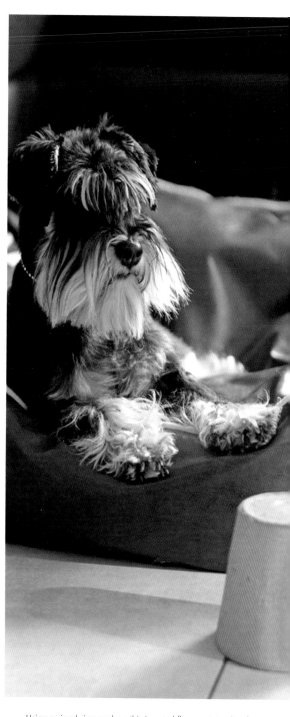

Using a visual sign, such as this inverted flowerpot, to signal to the dog that the owner is not available to interact with can be a very helpful tool in tackling many separation-related problems.

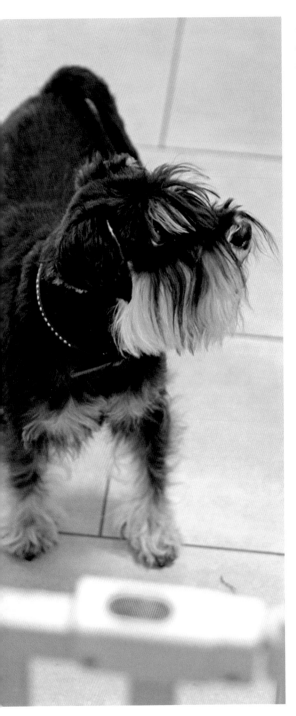

A correctly positioned and introduced indoor kennel or 'crate' can provide a secure haven for an anxious dog to go to and relax in when left alone.

Cassie has access to the kitchen and back corridor, hall, staircase and upper landing. The frosted glass front door is situated at the left of the staircase at the opposite end of the hall to the kitchen. Although there is a dog bed at the bottom of the stairs, this is where toys are kept and does not appear particularly comfortable. Stephen can be heard in the kitchen area preparing to leave; he doesn't speak to Cassie and although she moves around, she does not seem agitated. Stephen scatters a few choc-drops for Cassie by the front door to distract her before he leaves via the back door. She eats some of these and then watches the front door alertly as Stephen checks it's locked from the outside. His car can be seen moving away from the door. Cassie walks towards the kitchen (out of view), picking up the remainder of the choc-drops on the way.

The video recording reveals that after 42 seconds she whines once. Forty-eight seconds after that she howls. She vocalises a total of 98 times throughout the 1 h 2 min 30 sec video, and howling is more prevalent. This method of communication is reported to be used by dogs when seeking social contact (Serpell, 2000). About 9 minutes after Stephen leaves, she picks a Nylabone chew toy out of her bed and drops it again.

One of the most striking things about the recording is how extremely quiet the house is inside, although there is some occasional aircraft noise. Apart from barking and howling, Cassie seems relatively calm initially. However, as the howling continues she becomes more and more agitated, running upstairs sometimes, into the kitchen at other times and looking at the front door from time to time. On one occasion she jumps up near the letterbox. As her agitation grows she appears to become more aware of external noises, at one point she is alert and barking near the front door while looking towards the kitchen. She continues for about 4 minutes and seems apprehensive at this point. Although it is impossible to be sure, owing to the inability to observe her in the kitchen, Cassie seems to be constantly on the move for the whole of the video; this can be heard, if not seen. The house is near an airport and some distant aeroplane noise can be heard on the tape. Some of the louder plane noise seems to stimulate more persistent apprehensive barking from Cassie. Indeed one of the longer periods of howling and barking follows a loud plane passing overhead. The tape ends during a howl.

Observations during the Consultation

Cassie was at the door with Jane when I arrived for the consultation. She barked loudly as she followed me into the living room but didn't approach. I sat down and tossed her a treat and after a few repetitions she came and sat on the opposite end of the sofa and looked out of the window. From then on I was able to stroke her and scratch her under the chin.

Stephen was not able to be present owing to work commitments but he wanted to figure in the treatment plans. Throughout my visit Cassie did not seek Jane's attention in an overtly demanding way. However, she followed her closely everywhere and lay on the sofa in contact with her for much of the time, and Jane responded by stroking her. At other times Cassie lay on the floor in the living room, getting up if Jane moved. It was noticeable that, owing to the design of the house, in which all the downstairs internal doors are glass, she could observe everyone's location if she positioned herself in the hallway, which she did.

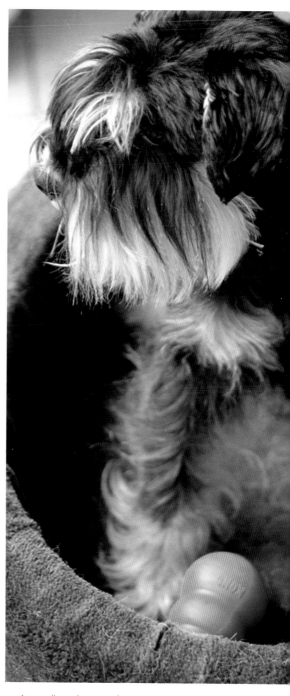

A treat-dispensing toy such as a Kong™ can be an excellent tool to help the anxious or bored dog to cope with social isolation, providing 'occupational therapy' in the form of interesting distraction and innately rewarding chewing opportunities.

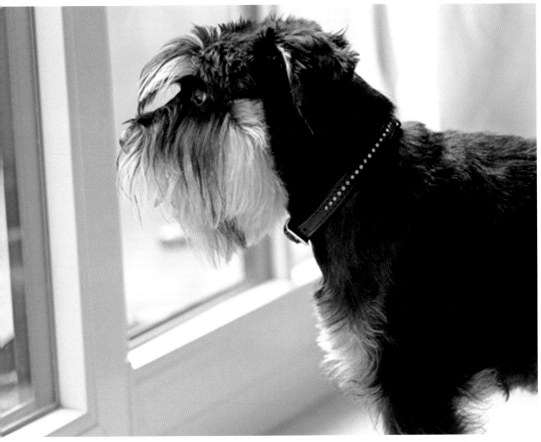

A dog that is stressed when left alone is likely to be more sensitive than usual to external stimuli. This often leads to further stress.

Possible Contributory Factors

Cassie came from a litter that was very well reared with regard to healthcare and attention and raised in the family home. This is of course excellent; however, early 'proofing' against a separation-related problem occurring in later life is unlikely to have been part of the rearing process. During weeks 3 to 5 it is beneficial for puppies to experience very short (a few seconds) periods of isolation away from their siblings and mother to prepare them for this experience (COAPE, 2012). Unless a breeder is aware of this, and the authors' experience is that very few breeders are, exposure to separa-

tion is unlikely to be a part of the early rearing process.

From the age of 7.5 weeks, Cassie has had company almost continuously except for irregular short periods when Stephen leaves for work. She is even clipped and groomed at home by Jane. In all probability, these combined factors have contributed to the current problem. Ideally, she would have been left alone for very short periods, either in a crate or a separated room, after she had settled into her new home, gradually increasing her time alone until she became habituated to it and it became inconsequential. When this had been achieved, the same desensitising process could be applied to the owners leaving the house.

Emotional Assessment

This is an estimation of the surge of feelings (good or bad) the Cassie might experience just before, during and just after engaging in the problem behaviour. Observing what could be seen of Cassie on the tape, she appeared to experience a range of emotions when isolated. She initially seemed to be disappointed and somewhat discontented – experiencing negative punishment on the removal of her owners (see Figure 20, point A). Consuming some of the choc-drops would suggest that she was not overly anxious at first. Early on, she could be described as somewhat bored. As the tape progressed, however, her emotional state underwent a change as she became more aroused and disinhibited (Figure 20, point B). She became more vigilant and then apprehensive, and more aware of, and then concerned about, the sounds she was then so acutely listening for. The overly effusive, lengthy greeting behaviour when her owners return can, in my opinion, be attributed to both elation (positive reinforcement – achieving a reward; Figure 20, point C) and relief (negative reinforcement – the 'bad thing', isolation, stops; Figure 20, point D).

Mood State Assessment

This is an estimation of how Cassie might feel during the rest of the day. Mood state can be defined as the average, day-to-day feelings of wellbeing, or as the feeling that is left after the ups and downs of the day have passed, and Cassie was described by Jane as being 'really laid back'. During my visit, once she settled down, she appeared somewhat lethargic. In fact, I thought she seemed unusually subdued for an 8-month-old dog. She had the demeanour of a much older dog. This is how she is much of the time. She spends long periods during the day looking out of the front window. The house is in a very quiet cul-de-sac where there is minimal activity. I would describe her mood as bored, bordering on discontented (see Figure 21).

Reinforcement Assessment

This is an investigation of exactly what factors, external and internal, are maintaining the behaviour problem, often in spite of many varied attempts to remove it. Cassie's behaviour is being reinforced by the return of her owners. Because the period of isolation is always relatively short, persistent vocalising is 'worthwhile' because it is so effective – Jane arrives home every time, probably when Cassie is still in an aroused state. The overwhelming relief she feels on Jane's return is highly rewarding after the increasing apprehension experienced while alone. The reward of the end of her isolation was proof in Cassie's mind that her strategy for dealing with the separation (vocalising) had succeeded and so would be the behaviour of choice in the future (see Figure 20). On top of this, barking and howling can be self-rewarding.

Hedonic Budget

The concept of representing and examining an animal's ethogram is not new (see Sambraus, 1998; Webster, 2005) and is used routinely in assessing the welfare of captive wild animals and domestic livestock. COAPE (2012) introduced the Hedonic Budget as part of the EMRA™ model as a measure of the behavioural characteristics of different types of dog. Information on the Standard Schnauzer from the Internet and books is sketchy but generally describes a dog that is protective, independent, spirited, friendly active and

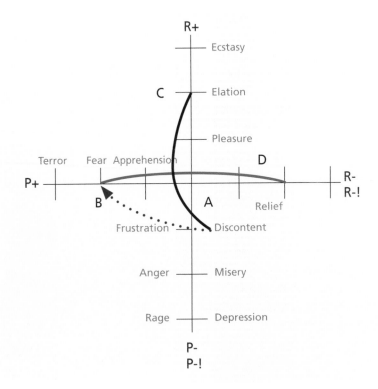

Figure 20: Assessment of Cassie's emotional state.

humorous. Schnauzers have been used as carriage dogs, dispatch carriers, ratters, retrievers, herders and search and rescue dogs. They were also the smallest breed to be used as a police dog in Germany, an excellent companion, protective of the home and family. They prefer people to other dogs (Rogers et al., 1996). Figure 22 shows our hypothesis of what the Hedonic Budget of a typical Schnauzer might be, compared with Cassie's prior to treatment.

Practical Interventions

After watching the video I felt that the amount of access Cassie had in the house when alone and her movement back and forwards in the hall and upstairs were contributing to her state of arousal

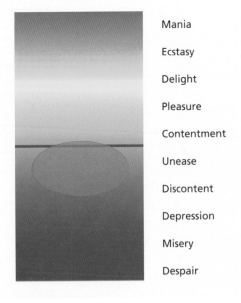

Mania

Ecstasy

Delight

Pleasure

Contentment

Unease

Discontent

Depression

Misery

Despair

Figure 21: Assessment of Cassie's mood state prior to behaviour therapy.

and apprehension. To try to alleviate this and to give her a feeling of security, I suggested the installation of a dog gate in the kitchen doorway. This limited Cassie's area of access to the medium-sized kitchen and side corridor. The frosted glass front door faces the clear glass kitchen door. As Cassie was aroused by seeing occasional ill-defined movement outside the bottom part of the front door, I suggested fitting a piece of cardboard over this to reduce the level of visual stimulation. A comfortable bed was to be placed in her new area containing her own bedtime quilt. Owing to the extreme quietness of the house itself, I suggested that a radio, set on a talk channel, should be left on at a low level to help mask external sounds. This would be turned on at least half an hour before the owner left, to prevent it becoming part of their departure routine.

Treatment Programme

Although Cassie's attention-seeking was mainly passive, I felt that she exhibited this behaviour often enough to consider the introduction of a 'signal of non-reward' (COAPE, 2012). The item to be used was a brightly coloured ceramic flower pot which I labelled 'Cassie's Pot'! When the pot was on view, Cassie was to receive no attention from her owners. When it was removed, attention could be freely given. Cassie would become familiar with the 'no attention' cue and would learn its significance, helping to increase her confidence while alone. Jane understood the importance of building up this technique very slowly, remaining in the same room as Cassie at first, gradually building up to very short absences in other rooms, to eventually going outside, always placing and removing the pot on her comings and goings. We discussed the importance of making departures and arrivals low key events,

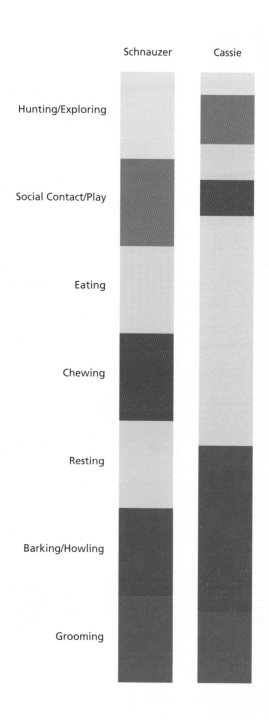

Figure 22: Cassie's Hedonic Budget compared with the ideal for a dog of her breed type and age.

delaying acknowledging Cassie until the non-reward signal had been removed.

The use of the dog gate was to be increased gradually also, incorporating the placing and removal of 'Cassie's Pot'. We discovered that she loved a Kong stuffed with food. Jane was to offer her a really tasty one as she left the kitchen pulling the gate gently to, and to remove it, as well as the pot, on her return. This technique utilises classical conditioning whereby Cassie will come to associate being alone with positive events, especially in the kitchen.

We discussed what other things we could do to improve upon Cassie's Hedonic Budget by encouraging her to exercise some of her intrinsic motor patterns (Coppinger and Coppinger, 2001). Introducing some interesting, breed-centred activities would enliven her generally and elevate her mood state. I had to be very careful at this point as I did not want to alienate Jane and Stephen by insinuating that she may have an unfulfilled life. We chatted about what Standard Schnauzers had been intended for, and decided that they have very diverse component needs, with apparently a bit of everything in their make-up. I explained that although Cassie had a wonderful life with devoted owners who clearly loved her and addressed her every need, there were some things we might do to encourage her to tap into her inherent doggishness and give her some dog fun. We brainstormed what we might do – it was important to encourage Jane to help to develop the plan so she could feel fully included in the process. We discussed Cassie's disinterest in her dry food. I suggested a change to a well-known hypoallergenic complete dry food for palatability and quality reasons. This was a great success and all Cassie's meals were now being eaten.

To stimulate Cassie's hunting/exploring side I suggested scattering some of her daily food allowance in the grass outside for her to find. We showed her how to search for some tasty treats and she had a great time finding the pieces. Most dogs love to chew and this was not something Cassie did. I suggested dipping Nylabone chew toys or sterilised bones into some left-over gravy and allowing them to dry for her to enjoy later. The sterilised bones could also be stuffed with tasty food. I had taken a Buster Cube feeding toy with me and Cassie played with this for a while with enthusiasm.

Stephen and Cassie love playing tug together and although dropping the item on cue had not yet been fully mastered, they were to continue this game. Cassie's enjoyment of chasing her ball was to be encouraged; teaching her to retrieve it and give it up would be addressed in training. Tying a piece of string round a soft toy for her to chase and pounce on and 'kill' was also suggested.

Cassie has two or three 20-minute walks a day, generally taking the same routes, however she is never allowed off the lead as her owners are afraid she will run off. Jane's dad allowed her off lead at the beach recently but everyone became anxious when she went off for a run! I felt that increasing Cassie's level of daily exercise would help to elevate her mood state. Exercise increases serotonergic activity and the release of endorphins, which also help to promote a feeling of wellbeing (Panksepp, 1998). It was agreed that Stephen would take Cassie for a longer walk nearer to his time of departure than was his habit to make sure she was tired when he left. This should ideally incorporate some off-lead running or, at the very least, some interactive play on a flexi-lead and include a variety of routes to provide new sights and smells.

I invited Jane to bring Cassie along to an advanced clicker class to allow her to meet regularly with other dogs and an empathic group who would be of great help in building her confidence around people. We dog walk after this class and this would present an ideal opportunity to allow

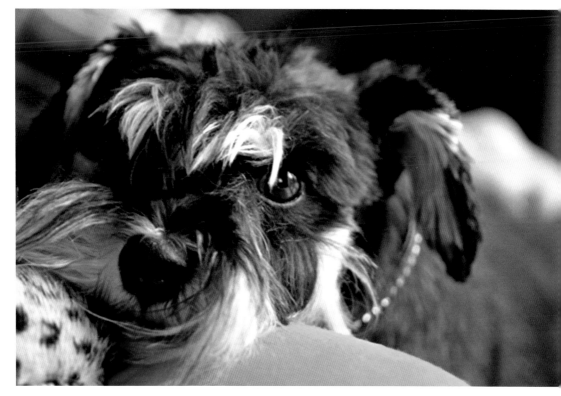

Even dogs that develop a very close relationship with their owners can learn how to cope calmly with social isolation if they are helped with careful early exposure to being on their own.

her some off-lead exercise with the group and provide support for Jane in taking that step. Jane mentioned that she would like to do more of the shaping and targeting exercises she had started with Cassie in the Junior Class. I asked her to show me how she was doing and suddenly, there was Cassie the loopy adolescent! She bounced around her target object (plastic cereal bowl) touching with her left and right paw, both on cue, followed her target stick and went off to sit on her carpet tile for a click and treat! The transformation was incredible, her mood instantly elevated and showed us the way to bringing further fun into Cassie's life. We also introduced her to 'dancing'. She was most enthusiastic about learning some basic dance steps and Jane and I had a lot of fun too! Some clicker work, particularly free

shaping, was to be introduced on a daily basis. Operant conditioning as applied in clicker training has a very positive effect in building confidence in dogs, I have found, partly as a consequence of the reinforcement they receive for working things out for themselves.

When Stephen left the house for work, he would hide at least two Kong toys in the kitchen and corridor area, leave the Buster Cube for her and secrete some dog treats here and there in corners and areas where damage would not be done with Cassie's searching technique. Although Stephen's departure routines did not seem to worry Cassie too much, he would vary them, performing some of his preparations, such as changing his shoes, at times not linked with departures. He would also ensure that the front door was locked well in advance of his leaving rather than checking it from the outside. From working slowly indoors using the Pot and Kong, Jane would progress very slowly towards stepping out of the back door for a few seconds and back in again, then closing the door momentarily when she was outside, gradually increasing her absences according to Cassie's level of tolerance. She was very aware that this would take time.

Both Jane and Stephen are highly motivated to try to help Cassie become comfortable on her own – not least because they would enjoy a trip to the cinema occasionally, something they haven't been able to do since she had joined the family! They are prepared to do everything possible to achieve a good outcome for her. The treatment plan would be passed on to Jane's parents who would do everything to help. At some later date, Cassie's distress on being left in the car alone would have to be addressed.

Follow-up

One week later: 'Cassie's Pot' was working well and was having the desired effect for short periods. She had become very enthusiastic about her Kongs and Buster Cube and used them when she was confined to the kitchen and Jane was elsewhere in the house. She was managing about 10 minutes of separation. She still followed Jane if she was not confined in the kitchen, but this was decreasing. A breakthrough for Jane came at the end of the week when she and Stephen had to attend a wedding for a whole day. A friend spent the day with Cassie and stayed the night. They arrived home very late and Jane looked in on her friend, who had gone to bed. Cassie was on the bed and although she was pleased to see Jane, she remained for most of the night with the sitter. Her greeting behaviour in general is less frantic

and stops sooner than before. Stephen was implementing his part of the plan and was enjoying taking various routes on walks. No off-lead exercise yet. Cassie has mastered 'Drop it'!

Two weeks later: Cassie was unconcerned about being left for extended periods of time in the kitchen while her owners are at home. Jane had noticed a marked difference in Cassie's general demeanour. She seemed more confident and was happy to lie in the living room while Jane went upstairs. She was still following her outside. Her greeting behaviour was very much improved. Jane's mum made the same comments when Cassie was with her. She still enjoys her Kongs and Buster Cube, has been dancing regularly (even for visitors!) and she's having a lot of fun with her clicker training tasks. Jane feels she seems more content. On the down side, Jane had to leave Cassie unexpectedly for an hour one day. She vocalised repeatedly on the tape but not at the same level as previously. Jane had left by the front door (they always use the back) and this had started Cassie barking before she'd even gone. Visitors arrive at the front and Cassie always barks, so I think this association has possibly influenced her behaviour. The back door will be used exclusively for the foreseeable future. Addition to training plan: Teach Cassie to sit quietly on her mat in the hall when visitors arrive. Otherwise, they are continuing with the programme and are very pleased with the results so far and have been able to step outside the back door for about 30 seconds. I explained to Jane that as Cassie becomes more familiar with the process, she may find that she will be able to accept time increases more easily.

Three weeks later: Jane has been leaving Cassie for short periods while she steps out via the back door. She has been able to close the door for about 5 minutes so far with no vocalising from Cassie. She is going to continue with this and now start to take a walk down the street. Cassie had an off-lead run on the beach at the weekend, chasing seagulls! Stephen has not had any night-shift work over this period. This is not a bad thing as it is giving her owners the opportunity to accustom Cassie to being left for lengthening periods before the challenging one. They're hoping to be able to take a quick trip to the supermarket soon! They'll let me know how it goes. Cassie's greeting behaviour has improved dramatically – one of the biggest changes – and she no longer follows her owners around the house.

Conclusion

Cassie presented with a moderately severe separation-related disorder, probably due to deficits in her early rearing with the breeder and to over-attentive owners, which in summary could be described as lack of isolation training. She had no strategies in place for 'surviving' being left alone. Setting achievable goals and providing support to the owners allowed them to start to progress towards improvement. Continued adherence to the treatment plan and including such activities such as joining the class and group dog walks should all help Cassie to develop into a well-adjusted dog.

Any deviation from homoeostasis must have an impact on behaviour, no matter how slight. Being emotionally discontented is as affecting to the individual as being depressed, differing only in degree. The clarity of the EMRA™ system opened a window onto the interface between emotion and mood where I could see it in action with Cassie. It demonstrated how crucial it is to look beyond the presenting problem and see the whole picture. The use of a video camera is an essential tool to this end; we would never have known the extent of Cassie's problem without it.

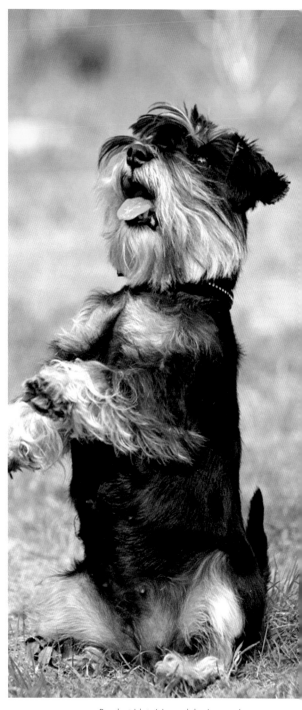

Regular trick training and shaping exercises are very helpful in elevating and maintaining a dog's general mood state.

Case History 6:
Aggressive behaviour

DOG:
Charlie, Rough Collie
AGE:
5 years
SEX:
Male (neutered)
PROBLEM:
Change in behaviour, biting

Charlie was obtained from a breeder at 5 months of age and he was castrated routinely at 6 months old. Since the death of her husband several years ago, Mrs E had lived alone with Charlie as her constant companion. Sixteen months prior to the initial consultation, Mrs E's two granddaughters, of 5 and 7 years old, came to live permanently with her, and subsequently Charlie had spent less time with his owner and found himself consequently rather excluded from family life.

A week prior to the initial consultation some relatives from Germany came to stay with Mrs E. They included young children and a mother who were afraid of dogs. During this time Charlie was completely excluded from the day-to-day activities of the family and was confined to the conservatory and not let into the rest of the house at all. This was because Charlie was a large boisterous dog and tended to jump up at the children and nip at them if they were running around or becoming excitable.

Problem History

While the owner's relatives from Germany were staying in her house, Charlie bit Mrs E when she tried to remove one of the children's toys from him. She reported that he had never bitten her or guarded objects before. She felt that his whole demeanour had changed, in that he was quieter in himself and grumpier. She reported that their relationship had deteriorated as she

A sudden denial of established pleasurable opportunities may contribute either to depressed behaviour or more reactive responses.

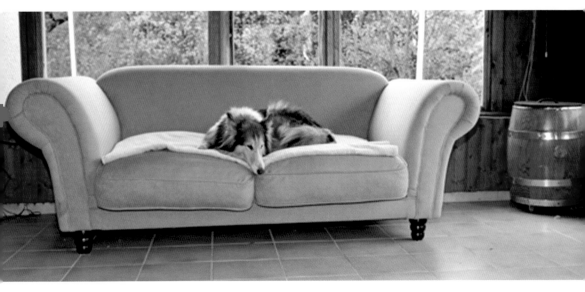

had become more hesitant around him, especially when handling and grooming. When Mrs E attempted to groom Charlie, he would stiffen, appear to threaten and so she would stop. She became concerned that there was a physical or medical cause behind Charlie's behaviour because there had been such a sudden change in his demeanour, and threatening and biting were so uncharacteristic for him. She was clearly very stressed and distressed by the whole situation. Her family from Germany were also very concerned about the dog's behaviour and so she was considering re-homing Charlie, a prospect that greatly upset her.

Observations and Practical Interventions

The bite from Charlie was visible on Mrs E's forearm, consisting of two small shallow puncture wounds and some bruising. It is important to assess the severity of any bites inflicted and also how much warning the dog gives before it bites to assess the safety of working with the dog, especially when children are in the household. Using O'Heare's (2004) classification of dog bites (see Figure 23), the bite Mrs E received was a level 3 bite as the puncture wounds were shallow and there was no shaking involved.

According to O'Heare (2004), dogs may be relatively easy to work with if they have inhibited bites at levels 1–3. Level 4 bites lack inhibition and are dangerous. Levels 5 and 6 are extremely dangerous and the risk of working with these dogs is usually too high to contemplate safe therapy, especially if the dog gives no warning prior to biting or there are multiple triggers (events) which cause it to bite.

In this case, the bite was in a very specific context of trying to remove an object from the dog, and Charlie growled a warning prior to biting.

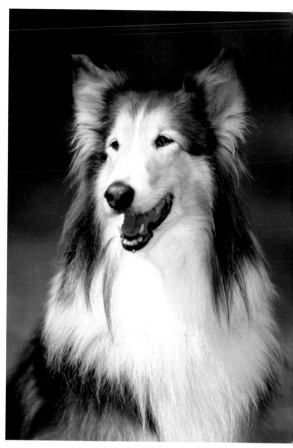

Social contact with people is an important element of the Hedonic Budget of all dogs.

When Charlie nipped at the grandchildren he did not make contact with them, but this was nonetheless a very serious issue that also needed addressing because the children are so young. The potential risks of working with Charlie and the alternative options of re-homing or euthanasia were discussed in depth. Mrs E wished to pursue the option of behavioural modification.

Classifications of canine aggression are outdated as they are usually contradictory and confusing, and trying to fit any case to such a classification is rather unhelpful in terms of organising an approach to treatment. For review see Lindsay (2001) and Mertens (2002).

The initial advice given to Mrs E was to remove Charlie temporarily from the situation at home until the relatives from Germany went home. This was to remove any risk of Charlie biting or scaring any of the children, to defuse the situation generally and to give Mrs E time to relax and consider objectively the options available to her. Charlie went to stay for a week with Mrs E's son who lives alone and whom Charlie knows well.

Level 1	Growls, shows teeth, barks, stares, snaps, no contact
Level 2	Single bite, saliva, no puncture
Level 3	Single bite, 1 to 4 punctures, half as deep or less as dog's canine
Level 4	Single bite, 1 to 4 punctures, greater than half as deep as dog's canine or shakes, there will be bruising evident within two days for very hard bites
Level 5	Multiple bites, greater than half as deep as dog's canine or shakes. Mauling
Level 6	Fatality

Figure 23: Severity of bites in bite-related injuries of humans (O'Heare, 2004).

A full physical examination revealed no abnormalities. Charlie accepted the examination without protest, remaining passive and appearing rather 'switched off', and made no attempt to interact at all, as would usually be expected from a dog undergoing examination. Routine biochemistry, haematology and electrolyte analysis was performed and no abnormalities found.

Emotional, Mood State and Reinforcement Assessment

As explained earlier in the case history of Bracken, the Cocker Spaniel, brain chemistry plays an important role in the Hedonic Budget of each dog. Following on from this discussion on breed type, Figure 24 shows an estimated Hedonic Budget for a 'Collie type', along with what Charlie's was estimated to be before and after treatment. As can be seen from the chart, there were many areas of rewarding stimulation and activity that were lacking in Charlie's life. One of particular importance was social contact – in this case with his owner. The lack of social contact that he experienced after the children arrived was in great contrast with the level of contact that he was used to when he lived at home with only Mrs E. Being shut away in the conservatory for long periods also denied him the opportunity to express other innate Collie behaviours, such as 'eye–stalk–chasing' the children (and nipping at their heels).

It would be logical to assume, therefore, that Charlie's mood state had become one of discontent bordering on depression (see Figure 25), and this would affect how he reacted in certain situations. So Charlie's emotional state (see Figure 26) when guarding a toy, or something else his owner

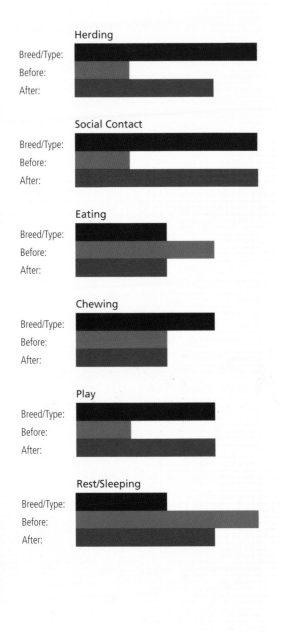

Herding

Breed/Type:
Before:
After:

Social Contact

Breed/Type:
Before:
After:

Eating

Breed/Type:
Before:
After:

Chewing

Breed/Type:
Before:
After:

Play

Breed/Type:
Before:
After:

Rest/Sleeping

Breed/Type:
Before:
After:

Figure 24: Ideal Hedonic Budget of an adult Collie in comparison with Charlie's.

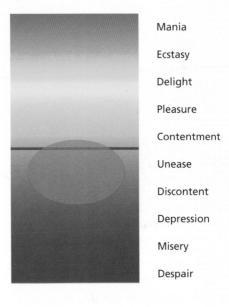

Mania

Ecstasy

Delight

Pleasure

Contentment

Unease

Discontent

Depression

Misery

Despair

Figure 25: Assessment of Charlie's mood state: initially (left), and after commencing treatment (right).

might try to take from him, quickly turned to one of frustration and possibly anger.

The reinforcement for the object guarding that Charlie showed was probably the relief of frustration that he experienced when his owner moved away and the reward of keeping the object he was guarding. This may also have become the case with grooming and handling as he had learned to apply a 'successful' strategy in other previous less challenging circumstances, but nonetheless with experiences that he would prefer to avoid.

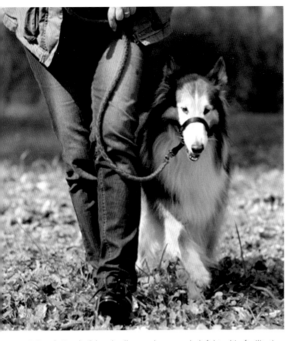

A Gentle Leader® head collar can be a very helpful tool in facilitating a relaxed, loose leash walk.

In conclusion Charlie had a depressed mood state due to an inadequate Hedonic Budget, leading to him to be overly reactive in situations of conflict, and to find relief for his frustration through inappropriate and potentially dangerous responses at certain times of emotional arousal.

Programme for Treatment

1. Hedonic Budget adjustment and restoration of mood state

The goal of treatment was to get Charlie from where he was (Figure 24, Estimated <u>before</u> for Charlie) to as close to the ideal for his type as practicable (Figure 24, Estimated normal for Rough Collie) and to restore his mood state (Figure 26). A routine was introduced, including

A dog's body language, facial expressions and speed and direction of movement all help in the assessment of their emotional state and overall mood state.

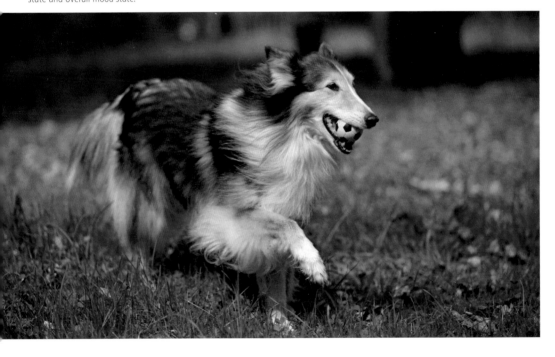

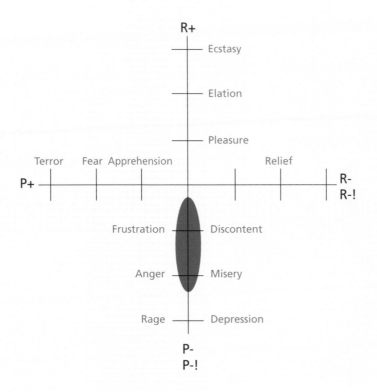

Figure 26: Assessment of Charlie's mood state after the commencement of behaviour therapy.

play sessions, training exercises, walks, interaction with the family and signalled quiet time, to achieve this.

Charlie had recently been excluded from the main areas of the house for the majority of the time and lived largely in the conservatory. With the arrival of her grandchildren, Mrs E has not had so much time with Charlie for walks or playing with him. She was worried about bringing Charlie into the house when her grandchildren were there because of his size and boisterousness. Child-gates were therefore introduced around the house to allow Charlie access to certain areas of

the house from the conservatory and to allow him to see the rest of the family and involve himself to a greater extent with what was going on in a controlled manner. The use of 'time out' was used to give Charlie down time if he became too excited around the children.

Once the children were back at school, Mrs E was able to bring Charlie into the house and spend much more time with him. Charlie had enjoyed playing ball games with Mrs E when younger and so these were re-introduced, giving Charlie an outlet for his eye–stalk–chase behaviour etc.

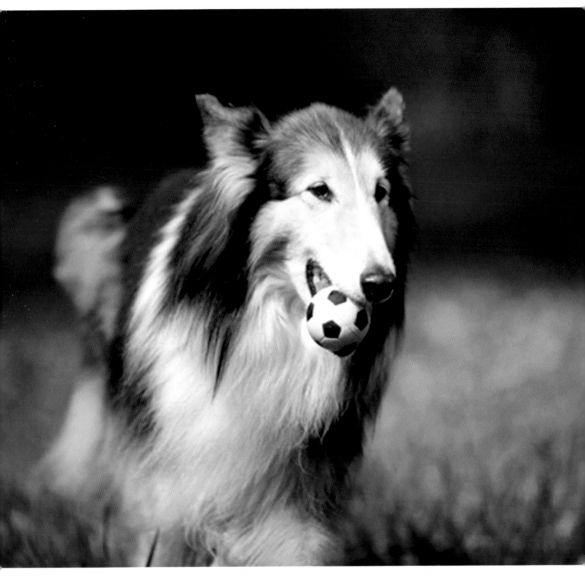

The additional frustration induced if toys are taken away from an already anxious dog may sometimes lead to unexpectedly aggressive behaviour.

Charlie was also trained to wear a Gentle Leader head collar so that Mrs E could take him for walks and play with him on a more regular basis. As a result he became much more attentive and responsive to her and became much more relaxed when put into the conservatory during rest periods.

2. Diet adjustment

Charlie was being fed a good quality complete dry food and it was decided to keep him on this. However, the once per day feeding regime was changed to twice a day to smooth any possible fluctuations in his blood glucose and the effect that this can have on behaviour (Strong, 1999). Part of his ration was also taken and used as reward treats during training sessions during the day.

3. Building Mrs E's confidence and applying the behaviour modification plan

Mrs E's confidence in Charlie had been compromised after the onset of his behaviour changes and so, in order to restore her trust, a specific plan was devised for both handling and grooming him using positive reinforcement training techniques to encourage him first to accept and then to learn to enjoy such contact, using a clicker (Kershaw, 1998). Charlie was fitted with a trailing indoor lead in the early stages of his treatment to give Mrs E a swift and safe means of control without coming into confrontation with him.

The greatest practical consideration in this case was safety, especially as there were children involved. The children were never left unattended with Charlie, and child gates helped in the management of the household. The children were taught how to react around the dog, for example standing still with their arms by their sides if ever he ran at them during games.

Treatment Outcome

Since the behavioural modification plan has been put into place, Mrs E has noticed a marked change in Charlie. She has found that he is much more alert and responsive to her; he seems to have more contrast in his behaviour between active times and rest periods, whereas before he spent much of his time just 'mooching'.

Mrs E is a very enthusiastic owner, who took readily to the idea of clicker training and the modification programme generally. Once the stress of the situation with her relatives from Germany had gone, and she started to 'see things from Charlie's point of view' (in her own words), she realised what a great impact on their lifestyle the grandchildren have had for both her and Charlie.

The grandchildren are much happier with Charlie now they have been helped to understand his behaviour towards them. They now do not feel that he is being 'nasty' to them, but that it is part of his natural herding behaviour. They are coping very well with the new instructions of how to react when Charlie runs at them – to stand still with their arms by their sides. They understand as well as they can, considering their ages, why they are doing this and how Charlie is responding.

As there are young children involved in the household, there will always be an element of management of the problem rather than a complete cure, as safety of the people involved is most important. This is currently being successfully achieved in this case.

The use of EMRA™ in Aggression Cases

The use of the EMRA™ model in treating aggression cases is useful and allows a more tailored approach for each dog rather than trying to pigeon-hole dogs into certain categories of aggression with more traditional and outdated classifications.

EMRA™ allows the dog to be assessed as an individual with differing motivations, emotions and reinforcements, which are all playing a part in creating and maintaining the behaviour. By understanding these motivations using the eye–stalk–chase sequences, and their emotions using the assessment models, the dog's needs can be far more adequately understood and met.

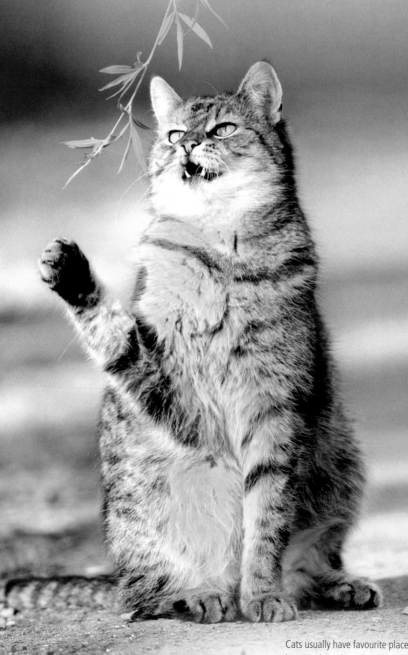

Bonus Chapter
EMRA™ and Cats

Cats usually have favourite places in their
homes where they play, rest and sunbathe.

CAT:
Neville, Domestic Shorthair
AGE:
6 years
SEX:
Male (neutered)
PROBLEM:
Indoor urine spraying

Introduction

Neville is a 6-year-old neutered male Domestic Shorthaired tabby cat, who is spraying urine indoors. He was reared with his littermates in an animal rescue centre in Ireland; the owner is not sure whether his mother or centre staff reared him. The litter were brought to a rescue centre in England at 16 weeks of age and Neville had already been neutered. He was then homed to his present owner at 5 months of age.

Neville had episodes of spraying since the owner took him home, but they were sporadic and at the same spray sites. However, Neville's spraying has become more regular over the last 18 months, with new sites and new items that include visitors' clothes, the owner's son's school bags and new toys.

The owner already had Max, a 2-year-old neutered male cat, when they took Neville on. The owner reported that Neville has always been a little nervous and shy but he did fit in well with Max and there has never been any aggression between them. The owner also introduced Poppy, a neutered female cat, 2 years after acquiring Neville. All the cats get on well and Neville gets on particularly well with Poppy, playing and sleeping together. The owner cannot recollect if Neville sprayed during this time.

A year later (2009) the owner acquired Jessie, a middle-aged spayed female Springer Spaniel. She settled straight away into the owner's home environment and the owner has not encountered any problems, for example aggression, between the pets.

The owner and her 11-year-old son live in a two-bedroom terraced house with a garden that is accessed from the kitchen. The kitchen door has a cat flap that the cats can access 24 hours a day. They are fed in the kitchen with separate bowls of dried food; however, as Jessie will eat the food, the bowls are moved if the cats are out and replaced if the cats come in. They will also eat from a bowl on the kitchen worktop; Neville in particular prefers to eat here. At night the owner shuts the lounge doors (see indoor layouts below), confining Jessie to the lounge and the cats to the kitchen overnight. Two cat beds, food and water are left on the floor in the kitchen.

Neville has been very healthy with only one incident where he required treatment for a tail injury and an overnight stay at the veterinary surgery. During the consultation, the owner mentioned that in 2007 the front of the house (the lounge and bedroom) had received extensive damage from heat and smoke because of a building that was on fire opposite their property. This resulted in windows exploding from the heat and smoke damage. The owner only had Max and Neville at this time, and Neville was not in the house during the fire. The owner had to move out for 24 hours but was able to shut the kitchen door so the cats could still gain their usual access to the kitchen from the cat flap where their food and beds are kept. Over the next few months the house had to undergo refurbishment and redecoration.

Observations

As is often the case with cats, Neville was not present during the consultation but the owner had taken a series of video clips of him over the course

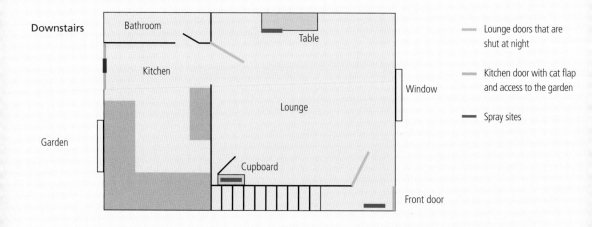

Figure 27a: Downstairs

of a week and I have based my approach to assessment and treatment on this evidence and the owner's account taken during consultation. The owner's main concerns are Neville's increase in spraying within the home and that she feels he is unhappy. The video clips showed various aspects of Neville's behaviour, his environment indoors and outside, and his interactions with the other pets in the home and with the owner.

Video 1 showed Neville's activity at one of four main spray sites. He is observed generally sniffing and investigating the cupboard. As he exits, he sprays a blue basket with characteristic marking behaviour, turning around, backing up to the spray site, his back slightly arched, and his tail quivers and vibrates (Bowen and Heath, 2005). He leaves a small volume of urine that has an oily appearance; the owner reported that there is also a distinct odour.

Neville's behaviour was characteristic of spray marking. Inappropriate urination, in this case spraying, is one of the main reasons cat owners seek behavioural consultation (Muller, 2010). Many behaviours that owners see as problematic are normal behaviours that are elicited because of conditions in which cats are kept (Rochlitz, 2000); however, developmental behaviour should also be considered as a possible reason why this normal behaviour has become a behavioural problem, and I will discuss this in my assessment.

The owner observed that Neville is more likely to spray when he first comes in from being outside and the areas involved tend to be the landing, in the cupboard if open, the plug sockets on the kitchen worktop, and furniture (see indoor layouts above). These are common sites that allow other cats to see and investigate them (Bowen

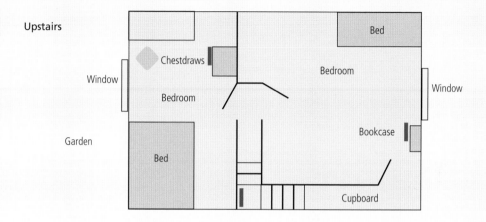

Figure 27b: Upstairs

and Heath, 2005, p.189). The owner reports that Neville's behaviour before he sprays indoors is relaxed; however, in Video 1, he had just come indoors from outside and in a quick glimpse, he is swishing his tail, perhaps indicating that he is agitated and in emotional conflict (Bowen and Heath, 2005). Neville also swishes his tail after spraying, perhaps indicating that he is still in a state of agitation and emotional conflict. I believe this is due to the presence of Jessie (the dog) in the doorway as Neville hesitates and then runs past, although it is not clear whether Jessie has been there since Neville came in.

In Video 2 we followed Neville leaving the house (afterwards, the owner found that he had sprayed on the landing), walking calmly but again swishing his tail and glancing back towards the house. He is then observed spraying a plant and jumping on to the fence where I believe he

sprayed again and then marked the fence by scratching it as well.

Neville's indoor environment in the lounge can be seen to be quite cluttered with toys, a normal situation that Neville has been used to since he was first homed. However, it is interesting that we see Jessie in her bed opposite this doorway and Neville's hesitance to pass through. I believe Neville is apprehensive at passing or being in close proximity to Jessie. Video 3 provided further evidence of this. Neville is seen trying to leave the kitchen via the window, almost pushing Poppy off the ledge. The owner commented that if the window were open, Neville would always enter or exit through it. We can hear Jessie's claws on the kitchen floor in the background, and so again I believe that her presence is the reason Neville does not want to leave through the door. Neville is subsequently seen outside sitting on the path swishing his tail, fairly calm but probably in a state of emotional conflict. As Poppy arrives with the typical greeting posture of her tail up with the tip bent, Jessie follows and Neville trots away and then sprays the fence. He remains in the garden but it is evident from his body posture that while Neville is not fearful, the degree of tail swishing does indicate that he is highly aroused and in a state of emotional conflict.

The owner has witnessed Neville spray in the garden at as many as three different spray sites in a matter of minutes. Neville shares the garden with the two other cats and the dog, but the owner is not aware of other cats having ever come into the garden and is only aware of one other house in the street that has a cat.

Owner Interaction

The owner acknowledges that Neville has always been shy and nervous and a bit of a loner. He rarely seeks physical attention as the other two cats do, for example rubbing around the owner's legs, sitting on laps or being stroked, and when other people are around he tends to leave or hide. The owner has never forced the issue because she accepted that this is how Neville is, however the owner does occasionally pick him up for a quick cuddle. The owner's reaction to Neville spraying has been to clean the sites using antibacterial cleaning wipes and she has, in the past, if she has caught him spraying, used a vocal reprimand and made a noise by clapping her hands together.

General Assessment

Urine marking is a normal behaviour used outdoors as a form of olfactory communication; some cats are quite social animals (although others less

so) but do maintain a certain amount of independence and, in particular, hunting is done alone. Olfactory communication is one form of marking territory. In unneutered cats the odour of sprayed urine is pungent and, as Bradshaw and Cameron-Beaumont (2000) state, this has prompted speculation that it carries other secretions from the preputial or anal glands and the strength of the odour reflects the success of the male and advertises his fitness as a mate. In relation to the female cat, if she is in oestrus the urine appears to carry important information about her sexual status (Bowen and Heath, 2005). The scent left by spraying can also minimise the risk of unfamiliar individuals encountering each other and potential confrontation.

It was thought that scent-marking was performed by confident cats trying to signal in order to deter competition from entering their territory, however it is now believed that marking indoors is an action of an insecure cat (Heath, 2007). The act of spraying is not only a way of marking territory or communicating the animal's status but can be performed when a cat feels angry or frustrated at some form of challenge, which helps to bring about some form of relief, in particular from stress.

A cat's territory is described by Heath (1993) as having its own home base, which is surrounded by the home range and beyond that the hunting territory. Cats usually scent-mark around the periphery of their territory. They use the home base for sleeping and eating, and the home range area for dozing, playing and sunbathing. With domesticated cats, the owner will normally determine the cats' territory, with the home base being the house, however this can be reduced even further in multi-cat/pet households to just a chair or cat bed. The home range is usually the garden. In densely populated neighbourhoods, the home base and garden can be quite small and

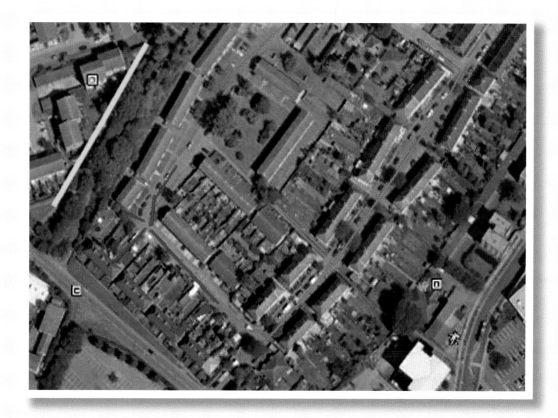

Figure 28:.Although cats are not seen within Neville's area, the aerial photograph demonstrates that whichever way he goes he is very likely to move into or come close to another cat's territory. Neighbours have also observed Neville spraying the tyres of any parked cars as he leaves the property and moves along the road.

if there is a high density of cats within a neighbourhood, hunting territories are very likely to overlap.

Neville's home base, range and hunting territory fit the description above. From observations gathered from the owner, her son and neighbours, the aerial photo shown in Figure 28 shows Neville's house (in blue) and surrounding neighbours. The blue line indicates the route he takes when he leaves the garden and the red lines indicate the neighbouring streets, where the owner is sure there are other cats but they are not seen in their area. The owner rarely sees Neville turning right and this is possibly due to Max, the older cat, taking this route and the presence of other cats in this territory. The yellow line indicates what used to be a disused railway line that has been made into a pedestrian walk/cycle way. The owner uses this for dog walking and has seen cats here too.

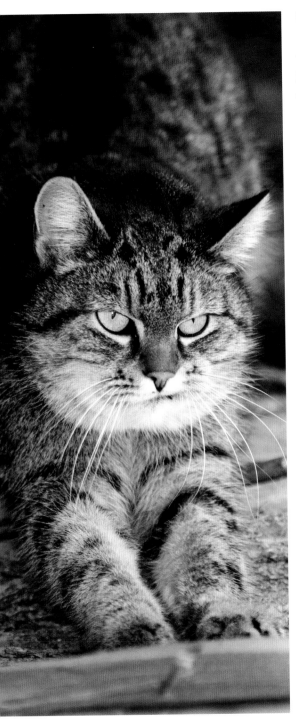

The EMRA™ System is ideal for the accurate assessment of behavioural problems in cats.

Emotional Assessment

To make an emotional assessment of Neville I will look at the observations and history gathered. I will also look at Neville's behavioural development, as I believe this may be the origin of Neville's behaviour problems. Little is known of Neville's life in Ireland, including, for example, whether his mother or centre staff reared his litter. Studies on the behavioural development of cats have found that there is a sensitive period for socialisation for kittens between the ages of 2 and 7 weeks (Turner, 2000) and kittens reared with their mother and littermates benefit from exposure to strong, biologically rich, suitable stimuli.

Further studies into the mother and kitten relationship from birth through to weaning have demonstrated how important this period is for the behavioural development of kittens. Weaning, as highlighted by Bateson (2000), is a period of major transition for kittens when a complete change from dependence on their mother to total independence occurs, and this involves a range of physiological and behavioural changes for both mother and kittens. The weaning process is an important part of the kittens' behavioural development, learning to accept not only different and more nutritious food but, importantly, the behavioural and emotional effects of frustration. It is thought that inappropriate weaning may predispose kittens to problems of aggression in adulthood (Neville, 1996).

Studies have indicated that cats suffer from stress when moved into catteries or rescue environments and this can, depending on the individual, last from a few days to weeks (Casey and Bradshaw, 2007). Cats' response to stress is highly adaptive and allows them to react rapidly and appropriately to a change in the external environment, however long-term exposure to an event can have a chronic negative impact on behaviour, health and welfare. Cats within a rescue centre are likely to be exposed to infectious diseases because of the sheer number of cats that pass through the centre, and the little that is known of their health or vaccination history. The rescue centre must ensure that exposure to disease, especially in the elderly and the very young, is reduced as much as possible. It is therefore in the cats' best interests if the rescue centre aims to reduce this long-term exposure and homes kittens as soon as possible.

During the early weeks of an average kitten's upbringing, it will be challenged by a huge number of environmental changes and social encounters. These will come from their littermates and mother and, later on, from other cats. Through maternal teaching and the development of exploratory behaviour, kittens gradually become habituated to commonly encountered noises and environmental stimuli (Neville, 1990). If we take the case of Neville, above, living in the rescue centre has determined his upbringing. Because of the risk of exposure to infectious diseases, it is unlikely that the physical environment the kittens were kept in allowed them to develop exploratory behaviour. They may have been exposed to an insufficient variety of stimuli to help them learn to deal with novelty and use their innate patterns of behaviour to learn which stimuli are potentially threatening and which are not.

This risk of exposure to infections within the rescue centre may also have had an impact on human contact. Studies have been carried out on the amount of handling given to kittens and the effect this has on socialisation with humans, and it has generally been found that the more handling a kitten receives, the friendlier it is towards humans (Turner, 2000). The centre would have been likely to reduce the risk of exposing kittens to infection by minimising the contact the mother

and kittens had with lots of different people during their first few weeks. This may go some way towards explaining why Neville does not actively seek interaction with people, including his owner.

If we consider Neville's environment over the last 3 to 4 years, it has undergone quite a few changes, including becoming more populated, with the introduction of two more pets (one of a different species), and extensive changes to the inside of the house through refurbishment, redecorating and a complete change-around of rooms.

Neville's way of dealing with these changes began with occasional marking. This I believe brought him some relief from the feelings of stress he was experiencing in an environment that exposed him to novel situations that he had not been exposed to during the sensitive period, or which he was innately prone to react to, perhaps by virtue of having a nervous character. When these periods of change or stressors finished, for example decorating, Neville's spraying reduced. However, the one stressor that has not disappeared is Jessie, and Neville's spraying has increased in his attempt to reassure himself. While urine spraying outdoors is usually performed quite calmly in order to maintain the integrity of a cat's territory, spraying indoors is often performed when a cat is at a high level of emotional arousal. Such spraying brings relief and reduces the state of arousal, albeit temporarily, and so the behaviour persists and probably often prevents other behaviour problems from developing.

Stress is a normal adaptive process essential for survival; cats' response to stress is highly adaptive and allows them to react rapidly and appropriately to a change in their external environments. Neville will disinhibit from his behavioural inhibition system (BIS) to deal with the changes within his environment. Through the stimulation of the hypothalamic–pituitary axis (HPA), noradrenaline and adrenaline will prepare the body to react

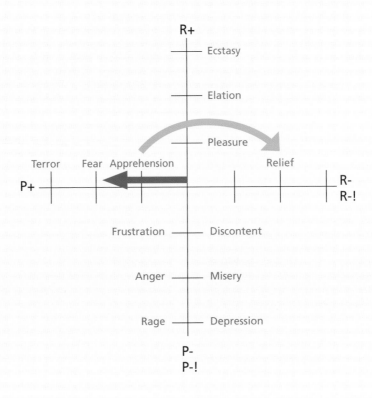

Figure 29: Assessment of Neville's emotional state.

rapidly to a possible threatening event, and stress response hormones will prime the amygdala to store a lasting memory of the event. Levels of dopamine, a neurochemical associated with the feelings of wellbeing, will fall. If an animal is unable to control, avoid or escape from the stressor, its stress response may become prolonged, it will be unable to disinhibit back to BIS, and this is harmful both emotionally and physically.

Neville resorts to spraying as the only way he knows of trying to surround himself with odours that will be comforting and bring some form of relief from the stressors within his environment. In Figure 29, the red arrow shows Neville's emotional state as he moves about his environment, and the green arrow indicates the emotional relief brought about by the act of spraying. Over time spraying no longer brings sufficient emotional relief and therefore he is now in a constant state of emotional arousal. The behaviour has not, however, escalated in frequency so it would appear currently to be at least partially effective as a coping mechanism.

Mood Assessment

Neville's mood state is one of unease and discontent because his attempt to deal with the stressor is no longer bringing him emotional relief.

Neville's Hedonic Budget is marked out of 5; his owner described Neville as a hunter regu-

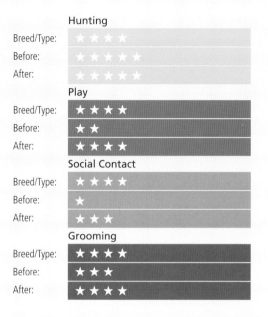

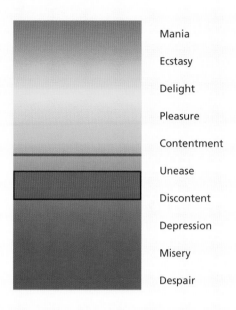

Figure 31: Mood State Assessment.

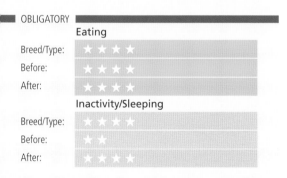

Figure 30: Neville's Hedonic Budget, before and after behaviour therapy, and in comparison with that of a typical cat of his age and type

larly bringing home birds and mice. During the consultation, the owner remarked that Neville does not like to interact or play with toys, however he does have a good relationship with Poppy and will play and sleep with her. Neville

does not have any problems associated with grooming. He has a healthy appetite and eats normally. Although the owner does report that she sees Neville asleep on her beds and chairs, she added that it can take him some time to settle and he does spend a lot of time under the bed or chair, another common feline coping strategy.

Reinforcement Assessment

Neville's behaviour is reinforced through the presences of the stressor and the owner's attempts to discourage Neville's spraying by use of cleaning and vocal commands. Neville is unable to feel relaxed with the original smells

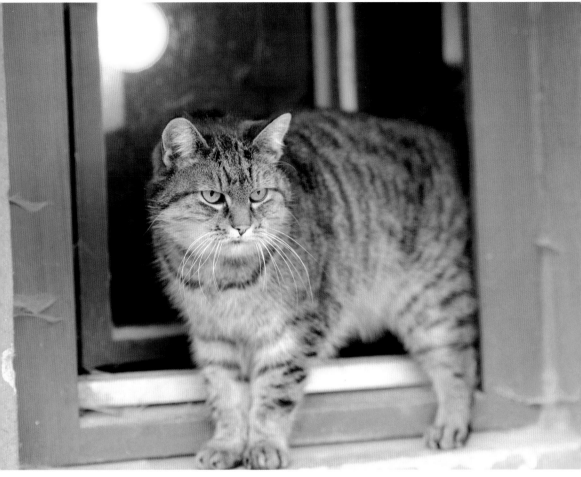

Spraying and urinating inside the home are the commonest behaviour problems in cats.

of his home environment and now must rely on his own efforts to ensure the marks remain fresh. Because he is in a constant state of arousal, the act of spraying is no longer providing Neville with emotional relief.

Treatment Plan

The aim of the treatment plan is to help reduce the stress Neville feels by improving his mood state to one of resting contentment. This will make him feel comfortable and content within his home environment and not feel the need to spray mark.

To achieve this, the first step involves robust cleaning of the spray sites, following the cleaning protocol (see later). It is important when cleaning that the products used are not scented or ammonia-based, because ammonia is a constituent of cat urine and may attract Neville back to mark. The use of alcohol (surgical spirit) helps break down fatty deposits in the urine (Heath, 2005. It is important to make these areas a source of comfort by placing food, beds or a synthetic phero-mone spray, Feliway® (CEVA), nearby. Feliway® is a synthetic analogue of the F3 fraction of the feline facial pheromone that is known as the familiarisation pheromone. It is believed to bring a feeling of security to cats in unfamiliar or stressful situations (Bowen and Heath, 2005).

Neville (1990) suggests that husbandry changes will help to fulfil instinctive behavioural needs, and the pheromone intervention will help the cat to be in a calmer state when exposed to emotionally arousing events. The owner should not use her past methods to deter Neville from spraying. The use of loud abrupt vocal reprimands and a handclap does not decrease the frequency or intensity of inappropriate behavior, but results in a marked emotional response and increased anxiety.

Neville likes to go upstairs where he can hide under the chairs or bed, however Jessie will sometimes go into the bedrooms. This could be the reason the owner has noticed that Neville finds it difficult to settle upstairs and has started spraying. Keeping Jessie downstairs by installing a baby gate, and introducing soft beds for Neville under the chairs, with his familiar smell, may encourage him to relax and settle here. The use of pheromones in these rooms may help him to find them a comfortable area for relaxation. Moving Jessie's bed from its present position next to the stairs will make Neville feel more confident about accessing this route to and from the bedrooms.

Ensuring that Jessie does not have access to the kitchen while the owner is out will allow Neville to feel more comfortable about coming in and out of the cat flap. Neville has sprayed the plug sockets on the worktop near to the window, which is his preferred access to and from the garden. Because of Neville's apprehension around Jessie, leaving via the cat flap if she is there causes him to become emotionally stressed.

To encourage Neville to accept interaction with his owner, observation of his body language is important, although it is worth noting that sometimes the opposite is better and the owner should be asked to leave the cat alone unless she is approached by the cat.

This is demonstrated in Video 4. The owner is seen communicating with Neville but, when he runs past, the owner's tone of voice is one of disappointment and concern that he does not seemed to be interested. On this footage, Neville is walking towards the kitchen relaxed with his tail held low but when the owner calls his name and tries to stroke him, he runs past and is swishing his tail as he goes to enter the kitchen – tail swishing indicates emotional conflict. The owner has not interpreted Neville's behaviour appropriately and, in subsequent footage, we see the owner pursue Neville and pick him up. He is swishing his tail but does not act aggressively towards the owner and when he is put back down his tail is held high in a greeting posture. A few moments later, we observe Neville spraying the shrub as he passes, perhaps an indication that he is still in a state of emotional arousal. The owner should observe Neville's body language and refrain from picking him up, but stroke him if he approaches with his tail held high in the greeting posture. This should, in time, allow Neville to feel relaxed when around the owner, encourage him to initiate contact and begin rubbing, which is a more pleasurable and relaxing way for cats to leave subtle scent markers.

The above treatments have been designed for easy practical implementation for the owner, however the wooden floors in the bedrooms are only painted and it is likely that any urine sprayed will have fallen between the floorboards, and scents will still be obvious to Neville, particularly when the heating goes on in the winter. It is advisable that wooden floors are cleaned and then varnished several times to form a seal and allow easy cleaning in the future but unfortunately this is not practical for the owner at this stage. The owner can also help by tidying the house where appropriate.

The main stressor for Neville is Jessie. As it is not practical to remove Jessie, the above plan is an attempt to make Neville's environment with Jessie less stressful by ensuring that there are areas in which Neville can get away from Jessie, and that access to these is made stress-free, perhaps by installing baby gates as dog-proof barriers at strategic doorways.

Outcome

The owner reported during the follow-up call that Neville had sprayed once but has not found alternative areas to spray. The owner has noticed a change in Neville's general behaviour as he appears to be more relaxed. The owner and her son are enjoying more contact with him now they are aware of his body language, and he is remaining to enjoy a stroke.

Prognosis

Cats with a history of indoor marking are likely to relapse, because marking is a normal behaviour. At some time in the future, situations outside the owner's control may create conditions that initiate a new bout of marking. It is very likely that this will be the case with Neville because this indoor marking behaviour has been going on for some time, caused by the stress he has felt within an ever-changing environment. Emotionally Neville has not been able to disinhibit to a state of relaxed wakefulness since Jessie came into the home environment.

It is hoped that the treatment plan described above will allow Neville to be able to feel relaxed and comfortable within his home environment. It does appear to be working, and the appropriate use of the pheromone spray Feliway® (CEVA) has been beneficial. Pharmacological drugs are used in cases of indoor marking and may be beneficial to Neville as this is a long-term ongoing problem. This will not help with the underlying cause, which is the continued presence of the stress trigger, but could be used in combination with a behavioural modification programme. Referral to a veterinary surgeon would be necessary for the prescription of behavioural medication.

Conclusion

This case has been very interesting and provided a few challenges in determining the most appropriate way to address Neville's behavioural problem. It has highlighted how important it is for kittens to experience appropriate socialisation during the sensitive period, particularly when they come from rescue centres that have to ensure that they are homed as soon as possible. It is worth noting that genetic factors could cause the same problem to arise in a cat that has gone through a 'perfect' early development programme, but this is usually impossible to examine or determine.

A review of housing and socialisation of mothers and kittens within rescue centres may help them adapt to a new home environment. One such area is early neutering, and this is becoming common practice. The Cat Group, a body of professional organisations dedicated to feline welfare, has produced a policy statement based on research regarding concerns about early neutering and the findings. Results of research into the implications for cat behaviour found no problems with behavioural development, however it is suggested that enough time is allowed between neutering, vaccination and homing to minimise stress.

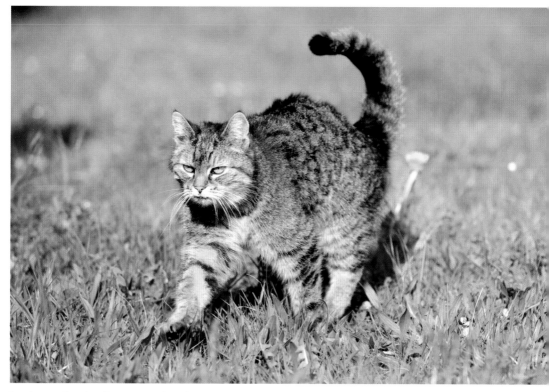

Cats that are allowed outdoors may not always be present during a behaviour consultation unless their owners are asked to keep them in beforehand, and even then may only rarely demonstrate their behaviour problems in company. Owners should be asked to film their cat's behaviour in the home and, if possible, the problem behaviour, in order to facilitate EMRA™ assessment and treatment.

I believe that Neville's problems have been generated by his lack of socialisation when young, however the problem has been ongoing since Neville was homed 6 years ago because initially his spraying was only occasional and in one or two areas that were easy to clean and so did not interfere with the day-to-day life of owner or cat. As such, a potential behavioural investigation into when and why he had sprayed was not considered.

With hindsight, Neville's history and the various studies into cat behaviour at our disposal, a different approach to introducing him to his new home may have prevented his lack of early socialisation in new and interesting environments from becoming emotionally stressful, and ultimately a behavioural problem. On the other hand, owners often do not fully understand the potential problems of multi-cat/pet households and assume they will all get along!

As Neville's indoor spraying had been occurring for a long time, I found the information regarding the history and all the changes proved rather confusing when trying to determine all the relevant possible influences on Neville's behaviour. The introduction of Jessie in 2009 is consistent with the 18-month period of increase in Neville's spraying and the owner noticing that he had become unhappy. The combination of key triggers – Jessie, and the change-around of bedrooms, an area Neville could go to that was away from the stressor – pushed Neville's emotional state beyond his coping threshold.

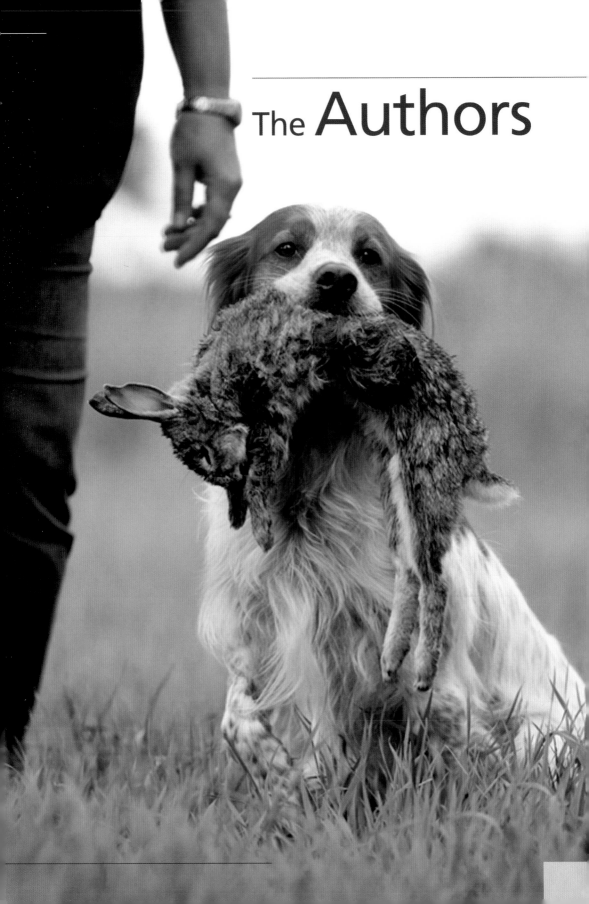

The Authors

Robert Falconer-Taylor BVetMed DipCABT MRCVS is a veterinarian and Partner in COAPE. He wrote or co-wrote and now tutors many of COAPE's courses. He also lectures and consults with animal and veterinary organisations, and is a frequent contributor to veterinary and companion animal media. He is a member of the Feline Advisory Bureau's Feline Behaviour Expert Panel and is actively involved with 'The Puppy Plan', a major collaboration between the Kennel Club and Dogs Trust canine rescue society in the UK. Robert is also a consultant to the pet industry, specifically engaged in the development of pet 'toys' designed to promote the welfare of pets and enhance their relationship with their owners.

Peter Neville Dhc BSc (Hons) is a founding Partner of COAPE. He became Clinical Professor at the Department of Veterinary Medicine, Miyazaki University, Japan in 2008 and Adjunct Full Professor at the Department of Animal Sciences, The Ohio State University, USA, in 2009. Peter is the author/co-author of 15 books, including the international bestsellers: 'Do Cats Need Shrinks?' and 'Do Dogs Need Shrinks?' He is the companion animal behaviour UK consultant to Purina Pet Care, a member of the Feline Advisory Bureau's Feline Behaviour Expert Panel and leads regular 'behind the scenes' safaris in Africa, studying the behaviour and ecology of African wild dogs and big cats. www.pneville.com

Val Strong MSc qualified as a medical scientist, went on to pursue a career in animal behaviour and training and has been a Partner in COAPE since 1997. She gained her MSc in Companion Animal Behaviour Counselling from the University of Southampton, UK, on the effects of diet on canine behaviour and training. She is one of the foremost experts in the assistance dog training industry and, having pioneered the training of sei-zure alert dogs to assist people suffering from epilepsy, she now lectures internationally on assistance dog training. She also has many years of experience in the training and rehabilitation of problem dogs and horses and has written a number of booklets on canine behaviour, diet and training. Val currently also heads a referral companion animal behaviour practice in the north of England.

Hannah Lyon BVetMed DipCABT MRCVS is a veterinary surgeon and Practitioner Member of the COAPE Association of Pet Behaviourists and Trainers (CAPBT) and is currently studying for her MSc in Clinical Animal Behaviour at the University of Lincoln, England. Hannah combines academic learning with practical training skills, being an Agility Club First Class Approved Instructor and a member of the Association of Pet Dog Trainers (APDT), for whom she regularly tutors courses. Hannah also runs the Behaviour Referral Service at the Ark House Veterinary Practice in Leighton Buzzard, Bedfordshire, UK, and provides a full range of behaviour assessments, consultations and rehabilitation classes. www.arkhousevets.co.uk

Billie Machell DipCABT gained the COAPE Diploma in 2005 and is an Affiliate Member of the COAPE Association of Pet Behaviourists and Trainers. Based in Aberdeenshire, Scotland, Positive Paws Puppy School provides Puppy Socialisation and Training Courses, Junior and Advanced Classes and One-to-One training and Billie integrates the EMRA™ approach into all her work with dogs. Billie is also a member of the UK Association of Pet Dog Trainers (APDT). www.positive-paws.com

Kirsty Peake DipCABT CABP MPSA is the current Chair of the COAPE Association of Pet Behaviourists and Trainers (www.capbt.org). She founded Pet Matters in 2000, which, involving three other CAPBT members, is now one of the

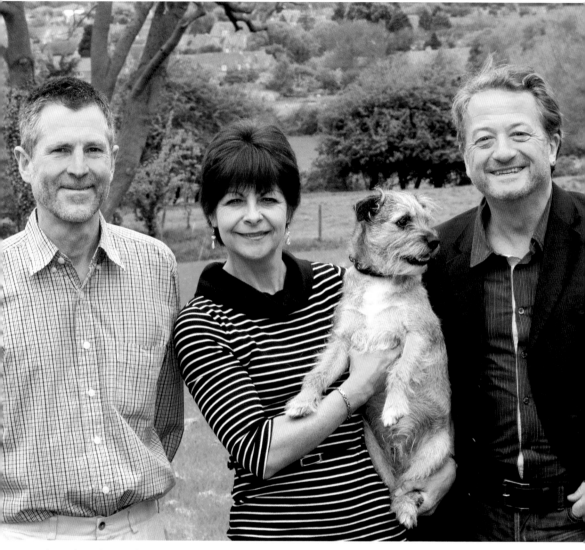

Authors Robert Falconer-Taylor, Val Strong with her Border Terrier, Dexter, and Peter Neville.

largest specifically qualified pet behaviour and training practices in south-west England. The practice offers behaviour problem referral services, a wide variety of dog training courses and workshops aimed at living in harmony with pets. Kirsty divides her time between practice and studying wolf behaviour while volunteering with research teams in Yellowstone National Park, USA. www.peakeservices.co.uk

Alison Rengert RVN DipCABT is a registered veterinary nurse with 23 years' experience of working with small animals both in veterinary practice and in pet re-homing centres. Alison gained her COAPE Diploma in 2011. She is currently establishing a behavioural training practice for both cats and dogs, but which will focus on the assessment and treatment of feline behaviour problems.

References and Further Reading

Bateson, Patrick:
Questions about cats: In The Domestic Cat,
The biology of its behavior.
Dennis C. Turner, Patrick Bateson (eds.)
12, 232. Cambridge University Press, 2000

Bernstein, Penny L.:
The human cat relationship
In The Welfare of cats, Irene
Rochlitz (ed.), 62. Springer, 2007

Blum, Kenneth/Cull, John G/Braverman,
Eric R./Comings, David E.:
Reward Deficiency Syndrome.
American Scientist 84, 132-145, 1996

Bowen, Jon/Heath, Sarah:
Basic tools in behavioural medicine.
In Behaviour problems in Small Animals.
Elsevier Saunders, 2005

Bradshaw, John W. S./
Cameron-Beaumont, Charlotte:
The signalling repertoire of the domestic cat
and its un-domesticated relatives. In The
Domestic Cat, The biology of its behaviour.
Dennis C. Turner, Patrick Bateson (eds.).
Cambridge University Press, 2000

Casey, Rachel A./Bradshaw John W. S.:
The assessment of welfare In
The Welfare of cats.
Irene Rochlitz (Hrsg.), 28. Springer, 2007

COAPE:
Course Notes, Diploma, Practical Aspects of
Companion Animal Behaviour and Training.
Ross-shire, 2012

Coppinger, Ray und Lorna:
Dogs: A Startling New Understanding of
Canine Origin, Behavior and Evolution.
New York: Scribner, 2001

Goleman, Daniel: Emotional Intelligence.
London: Bloomsbury Publishing, 1996

Heath, Sarah:
Why does my cat?.
Blaina: 62 Creative Print & Design, 1993

Heath, Sarah:
Behavioural problems and welfare.
In The Welfare of cats,
Irene Rochlitz (ed.) 106. Springer, 2007

Kershaw, Elizabeth:
Go Click! An Introduction
to Clicker Training.
Pet Behaviour Centre, 1998

Koob, George F./Le Moal, Michel:
Drug Abuse: Hedonic Homoeostatic
Dysregulation. Science 278, 52-58, 1997

Le Doux, Joseph:
The Emotional Brain.
London: Weidenfeld and Nicholson, 1998

Leung, L. Stan/Ma, Jingyi/
McLachlan, Richard S.:
Behaviors induced or disrupted
by complex partial seizures.
Neuroscience and Biobehavioral Reviews 24,
763-775, 2000

Lindsay, Steven R.:
Handbook of Applied Dog Behavior
and Training.
Ames: Iowa State University Press, 2000

Mendl, Michael/Hardcourt, Robert:
Individuality in the domestic cat: origins,
development and stability In: The Domestic
Cat, The biology of its behavior.
Dennis C. Turner, Patrick Bateson (Hrsg.). 4, 54.
Cambridge University Press, 2000

Mertens, Petra: Canine Aggression. In: BSAVA
Manual of Canine and Feline Behavioural
Medicine, 1. Auflage,
Horwitz, Debra F./Mills, Daniel S./Heath, Sarah/
BSAVA (Hrsg.), Gloucester, UK. 119-127, 2002

Mills, Daniel S.:
Medical paradigms for the study of problem
behaviour: a critical review.
Applied Animal Behaviour Science 81, 265-277,
2003

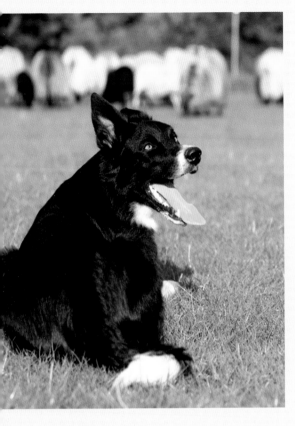

Muller, Gerard:
Canine and feline behavioural matters.
In Veterinary Focus 20(1), 2010

Naranjo, Claudio A./Tremblay, Lescia K./Busto, Usoa E.:
The role of the brain reward system in depression. Prog. Neuro-Pyschopharmacol. & Biol. Pyschiatr. 25, 781-823, 2001

Neville, Peter:
Cat Behaviour Explained,
29. Mackays of Chatham, 1990

Neville, Peter:
The behavioural impact of weaning on cats and dogs.
Veterinary Annual 36, 98-108, 1996

O'Heare, James:
The Canine Aggression Workbook. 3. Auflage,
Ottawa: DogPsych, 2004

Panksepp, Jaak:
Affective Neuroscience.
Oxford: Oxford University Press, 1998

Rochlitz, Irene:
The Feline welfare issues In: The Domestic Cat,
The biology of its behavior. Dennis C. Turner,
Patrick Bateson (Hrsg.). 11, 220. Cambridge
University Press, 2000

Rogers Clark, Anne/ Brace Andrew H. (Hrsg):
The International Encyclopedia of Dogs.
London: B.T. Batsford Ltd., 1996

Rolls, Edmund T.:
The Brain and Emotion.
Oxford: Oxford University Press, 1999

Sambraus, Hans:
Applied ethology - its task and
limits in veterinary practice.
Applied Animal Behaviour Science, 59(1-3),
39-48, 1998

Serpell, James (Hrsg.):
The Domestic Dog. Cambridge:
Cambridge University Press, 2000

Strong, Val:
The Dogs Dinner.
The Implications of Diet on Behaviour.
New York: Alpha Books, 1999

Turner, Dennis C.:
The human cat relationship . In: The
Domestic Cat, The biology of its behavior.
Dennis C. Turner, Patrick Bateson (Hrsg.). 12,
232. Cambridge University Press, 2000

The Cat group. Grundsatzerklärungen:
URL: http://www.fabcats.org/cat_group/
policy_statements/neut.html 18.08.11

Walker, Robin/Fisher, John/Neville, Peter F.:
The treatment of phobias in the dog. Applied
Animal Behaviour Science 52, 275-289, 1997

Webster, John:
Animal Welfare: Limping towards Eden.
Oxford: Blackwell Publishing, 2005

Website des britischen Kennel Club
www.the-kennel-club.org.uk

Index

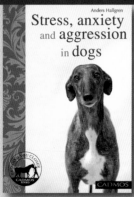
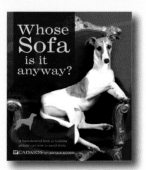
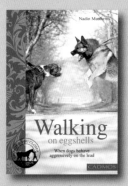
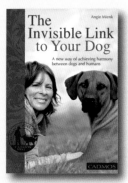